# FOR THOSE WE LOVE

## A Spiritual Perspective on AIDS

# FOR THOSE WE LOVE

## A Spiritual Perspective on AIDS

Second Edition, Expanded

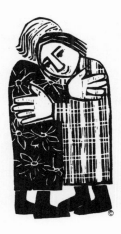

AIDS Ministry Program
The Archdiocese of Saint Paul and Minneapolis

The Pilgrim Press
Cleveland, Ohio

*Graphic design and typesetting for first edition by:*
*Heidi Waldmann, Choice Words, St. Paul, Minnesota*

Scripture quotations, except as noted below, are taken from the
*New American Bible with Revised New Testament,* copyright © 1986,
Confraternity of Christian Doctrine, Washington, D.C., and are used
with permission. All rights reserved.

Micah 6:8b is taken from *The Holy Bible, New International Version,*
copyright © 1978 by New York International Bible Society

Library of Congress Cataloging-in-Publication Data

For those we love: a spiritual perspective on AIDS/AIDS Ministry
    Program, the Archdiocese of Saint Paul and Minneapolis.—2nd
    ed., expanded
        p. cm.
     ISBN 0-8298-0919-8: $8.95
      1. AIDS (Disease)—Patients—Religious life. 2. AIDS (Disease)
—Religious aspects—Catholic Church. 3. Caregivers—Religious
life. 4. Catholic Church—Membership. I. Catholic Church.
Archdiocese of St. Paul and Minneapolis. AIDS Ministry Program.
BX2347.8.A52F67    1991
248.8'6—dc20                         91-38772
                                       CIP

This book is printed on acid-free paper

Printed in the United States of America

Second Edition, Expanded
10  9  8  7  6  5  4  3  2  1
The Pilgrim Press, Cleveland, Ohio

## Dedication:

For you who live with the illness of AIDS, for those you love, and for all those who care about your every need.

To

Brother Louis Blenkner, OSB
St. John's University, Collegeville, Minnesota

who stands as a model for the Christian caregiver

and with gratitude to the Archdiocese of Saint Paul and Minneapolis for the gentle and faithful presence of their AIDS ministry volunteers.

With special thanks to all who have contributed so much of themselves to make this book a reality:

| | | |
|---|---|---|
| Kathy Briggs | Bill Kummer | Dee Ready |
| Mary Ann Carolin | Bill Lee | Carol Richer |
| Kevin Daly | Joanne Lucid | Nan Ross |
| Jim DeBruycker | Helen Major | Katie Schulte |
| Rose Diestler | Lons Mass | Martin Shallbetter |
| Keith Gann | Sharon Muir | *Star Tribune* |
| Darlene Gray | Hannah Ofsthun | Heidi Waldmann |
| Ron Joki | Mark O'Leary | Ron Wilson |
| Jim Klobuchar | Lydia Pizel | Carl Winkles |
| | Tim Power | |

# Contents

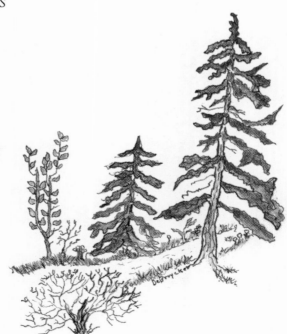

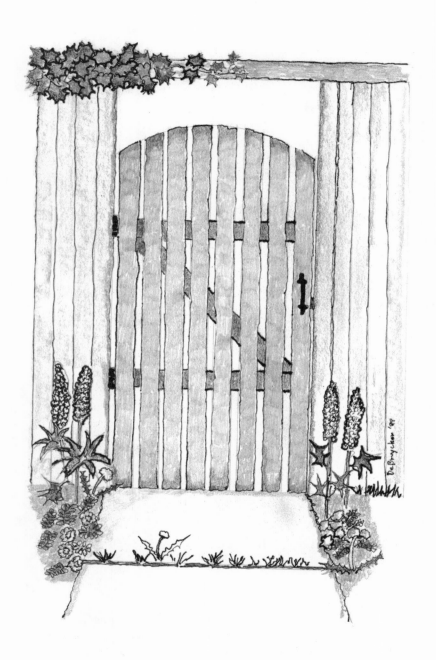

# Introduction

## How Do We Walk Together?

THE AIDS EPIDEMIC has certainly brought about tremendous pain and anguish for a great many members of the human family. It poses many serious dilemmas for us—social, political and medical, to name but a few. This handbook focuses primarily on another aspect of AIDS that is often overlooked and yet is ultimately, perhaps, its greatest dilemma—spirituality.

A spiritual response can be a critical part of the lives of persons living with AIDS. Whether we embrace more traditional forms or find New Age ideas helpful, the intent is the same: we hope to find some kind of spiritual peace with AIDS.

A simple definition of spirituality suggests that, although broken and fragmented, we can come to peace with our brokenness and come to find acceptance in our own imperfection. From this more peaceful state of mind, creativity and the ability to love unselfishly—which go hand in hand—can come much easier to us. Acceptance, faith, forgiveness, peace and love are traits that define this spirituality. It is no coincidence that these same characteristics always appear in persons who achieve an unexpected healing of a terminal or serious illness of the mind, body or spirit.

At the heart of these journeys of healing is the choice to remain within the physical experience of life. The strongest anchors to the physical experience of life are love and a belief that our lives are significant and meaningful. The feeling that our lives are valueless, meaningless and loveless fuels the damaging power of this disease. And yet, value, meaning and love cannot be created upon demand. They emerge from within our being when we are ready to seek them. For many of us, prayer, meditation and listening to one's inner guidance can be very strong medicines. Many have found that prayer and introspective thought ignite a level of courage and inner wisdom within themselves from which springs forth the natural healing capacity of the human spirit. Most of us believe in life after death and in God. An activation of those beliefs and of a sense of purpose is the most important factor anyone can use to create health and healing. In a time of great despair, one simple question may serve to initiate hope: "What can I learn from this experience in order to become a more spiritually mature person?"

There is no doubt that persons living with AIDS have a great need for support, care and, most of all, friendship. It is the small gesture, the quiet moment and the shared time that give meaning to a person's day as we walk this path together. As the relationship grows between the spiritual caregiver and the person with AIDS, both individuals grow and flourish—nurturing themselves and each other, learning, sharing and reaping the rewards of learning about oneself and, ultimately, empowering and being empowered. Inevitably, the relationship reaches a crux of frustration and an overwhelming sense of uselessness and fear; it is at this very time when our faith alone will carry us.

There are many things that we can do and will do. There is nothing magical that is required of us as we enter into or pursue this sacred relationship that is such a powerful sign of Christ's presence among us. And if we truly want to achieve some spiritual peace with AIDS, these relationships as friends are crucial. When we give up trying to make God's ways seem humanly reasonable, then it is precisely through our acts of loving, of listening, of tending the sick and dying, of comforting the bereaved that we spiritually feed and heal one another, and in so doing bring in the Kingdom.

**This book offers you a composite of reflections from people who, like you, live with the AIDS virus. Like you, each of these people has encountered both fear and hope. Each has known both the isolation of silence and the joy of sharing. Each has experienced both the grief of lost dreams and the exhilaration of newfound strength. Use this book to ask your own questions, to write your own answers, and to discover your own feelings. Agree or disagree with what you read. Seek the help of others; read a listed book; make your own decisions; cope with the life you find yourself living today.**

For today brings you the opportunity to feel, to hear, to see, to express love and compassion. Before illness, you may have assigned these activities to a distant someday. That someday is now. Reach out now.

May these words and shared experiences become a source of courage, faith, love, and spiritual well-being for you.

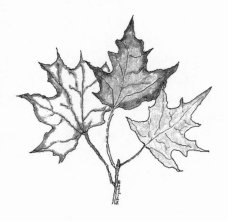

## Healing and Hope

*In beginning the journey toward hope and healing, let us listen to a person who has lived with AIDS for five years and has struggled with many of the issues.*

FOR ME, HEALING INVOLVES a balance of body, mind, heart, and spirit. I must let go of my goals so that my life can flow in the direction I'm going. I must trust unknown forces, such as the universe, to bring me to a safe haven. I must hand over the process of my life to a higher power. When I do these things, I have enough energy, strength, and courage to take responsibility for those things in my life over which I do have control, such as how well I care for my body, stimulate my mind, express my heart, and nurture my spirit. On a day-to-day basis, these actions enhance my life in spite of my losses and pain. Daily I let go of what I've lost or what hurts and concentrate on the day-by-day process of life in a balanced way. When I do this, hope, which is the sustainer and healer of life, blossoms forth in me.

**Am I isolated with my own secret pain? In what way?**

*Have I had anyone with whom to talk? Who?*

*Right now, where am I in my pain?*

*Would having a buddy be helpful now?*

*Who provides me with laughter and support and caring right now?*

*Right now, what can I do about what I am feeling?*

Perhaps all your heart can discover about your feelings is that you want to give an agonized cry to express your powerlessness. Would any of the suggestions on the following pages be helpful to you?

# Would prayer be helpful now?

*What things bring you peace of mind, what things are restful for you, what helps to ease your burdens? Sometimes you may want to be alone, sometimes you may want companionship. What follows are suggestions coming from other people who have walked this path and have found peace and comfort in scripture, in poetry, in music, in books.*

## Scripture

### Acceptance

"My father, if it is possible, let this cup pass from me; yet, not as I will but as you will." (Matthew 26:39)

Luke 2:29-32 (Simeon's prayer, "Nunc Dimittis")

Luke 15 (Parables of the Lost Sheep, Lost Coin, and Lost Son)

Luke 19:1-9 (Zacchaeus)

### Anger

Matthew 23 (Denunciation of the Scribes and Pharisees)

## Comfort

Who will bring a charge against God's chosen ones? It is God who acquits us. Who will condemn? It is Christ [Jesus] who died, rather, was raised, who also is at the right hand of God, who indeed intercedes for us. What will separate us from the love of Christ? Will anguish, or distress, or persecution, or famine, or nakedness, or peril, or the sword? As it is written:

"For your sake we are being slain all the day;
we are looked upon as sheep to be slaughtered."

No, in all these things we conquer overwhelmingly through him who loved us. For I am convinced that neither death, nor life, nor angels, nor principalities, nor present things, nor future things, nor powers, nor height, nor depth, nor any other creature will be able to separate us from the love of God in Christ Jesus our Lord. (Romans 8:33-39)

Isaiah 55 ("Come to the Water")

Luke 1:76-79 (The Canticle of Zechariah)

## Death

Behold, I tell you a mystery. We shall not all fall asleep, but we all will be changed, in an instant, in the blink of an eye, at the last trumpet. For the trumpet will sound, the dead will be raised incorruptible, and we shall be changed. For this which is corruptible must clothe itself with incorruptibility, and this which is mortal must clothe itself with immortality. And when this which is corruptible clothes itself with incorruptibility and this which is mortal clothes itself with immortality, then the word that is written shall come about.

"Death is swallowed up in victory.
Where, O death, is your victory?
Where, O death, is your sting?"
(1 Corinthians 15:51-55)

2 Samuel 14:14

Wisdom 3:1-9

Isaiah 25:6-9

Psalm 23

Revelations 21:1-7

## Depression

Psalm 102:1-13

John 14:16-19

## Doubt

...I do believe. Help my unbelief! (Mark 9:24b)

John 20:24-29

Matthew 8:5-13 (The Healing of the Centurion's Servant)

Mark 4:35-41 (The Calming of a Storm at Sea)

## Exhaustion and Burden

Come to me, all you who labor and are burdened, and I will give you rest. Take my yoke upon you and learn from me, for I am meek and humble of heart; and you will find rest for yourselves. For my yoke is easy, and my burden light. (Matthew 11:28-30)

Psalm 13

Psalm 144

Matthew 5:1-12 (Beatitudes)

Luke 10:38-41 (Martha and Mary)

## Faith

Matthew 9:20-22

Romans 5:1-5

**Fear**

> Fear not, I am with you;
>> be not dismayed; I am your God.
> I will strengthen you, and help you,
>> and uphold you with my right hand of justice.
>> (Isaiah 41:10)

Psalm 91 ("Eagle's Wings")

Isaiah 43:1b-3 ("Be Not Afraid")

Matthew 8:23-27

**Forgiveness**

Psalm 139

Matthew 9:1-8

Romans 14:1-13

Luke 7:36-50 (Jesus Anointed with Perfume)

**Guilt**

> And what does the Lord require of you? To act justly
> and to love mercy and to walk humbly with your God.
> (Micah 6:8b, NIV)

Psalm 32

**Hope**

John 11:1-44 (The Raising of Lazarus from the Dead)

Romans 8:22-27

1 Thessalonians 4:13-18

**Loneliness**

> I will not leave you orphans; I will come to you.
> In a little while the world will no longer see me,
> but you will see me, because I live and you will live.
> (John 14:18)

Psalm 22:20-21

John 16:32-33

**Pain of Loss**

> My God, my God, why have you forsaken me,
>      far from my prayer, from the words of my cry?
> O my God, I cry out by day, and you answer not;
>      by night, and there is no relief for me.
>      (Psalm 22:1-3)

Luke 22:39-46 (The Agony in the Garden)

**Patience**

Psalm 130

Isaiah 40:28-31

Colossians 1:9-14

**Stress**

> Come to me, all you who labor and are burdened,
> and I will give you rest. (Matthew 11:28)

Psalm 142

Luke 22:39-46 (The Agony in the Garden)

**Tears**

Psalm 31

Psalm 42:1-4

Ecclesiastes 3:1-8

John 11:17-36

**Trust**

> Jesus, remember me when you come into your kingdom. He replied to him, "Amen, I say to you, today you will be with me in Paradise." (Luke 23:42-43)

Psalm 86:1-13

Psalm 139:1-18

Matthew 7:7-11

*What prayers are helping me right now?*

# Would reading poetry be helpful now?

**Death**

"Do Not Go Gentle into That Good Night" by Dylan Thomas

"After Great Pain a Formal Feeling Comes" by Emily Dickinson

"Death, Be Not Proud" by John Donne

**Faithfulness**

"Dover Beach" by Matthew Arnold

**Hope**

"Hope" and "Abandonment" from *God Speaks* by Charles Peguy

"Hope Is the Thing with Feathers" by Emily Dickinson

"Stopping by Woods on a Snowy Evening" by Robert Frost

**Laughter**

"Elegy on the Death of a Mad Dog" by Oliver Goldsmith

"The Cremation of Sam McGee" by Robert Service

"The Twins" by Henry S. Leigh

**Life**

"Crystal Moment" by Robert P. Tristram Coffin

**Love**

"The Thought" by Edward Herbert, Lord of Cherbury

"Sonnet 116" by Shakespeare

"Sonnet 43" by Elizabeth Barrett Browning

**Memories**

"Piano" by D. H. Lawrence

"Before the Light Fades" by Frances Bellerby

**Steadfastness**

"Choose Something like a Star" by Robert Frost

**Praise**

"Pied Beauty" by Gerard Manley Hopkins

**Thankfulness**

"Apologia" by Phyllis McGinley

"i thank You God for most this amazing" by e.e. cummings

*What poems are helping me right now?*

# Would listening to music be helpful now?

*The Four Seasons* by Vivaldi

Music by Kitaro

Music by George Winston

*The Messiah* by Handel

*Canon* by Pachelbel

Music by John Michael Talbot

*Symphony No. 9* by Beethoven


**What music is helping me right now?**

*Have I read something helpful recently?*

*Am I aware of the resources in my community?*

**Minnesota:**

AIDS Ministry Program
   612/337-4345 (24-hour answering)

Minnesota AIDS Project (MAP)
   Seven-county metro area  612/870-0700
   Greater Minnesota 800/248-AIDS (800/248-2437)

AIDS Interfaith Council of Minnesota (AICM)
   612/870-7773

**National:**

National AIDS Hotline: 800/342-AIDS (800/342-2437)

National Spanish AIDS Hotline: 800/344-SIDA
   (800/344-7432)

National Catholic AIDS Network: 202/387-8017

AIDS National Interfaith Network: 212/239-8700

(See Directory of People, Places, and Other Resources beginning on page 113.)

## What am I doing to handle stress?

### Exercise and recreation

### Nutrition

### Meditation

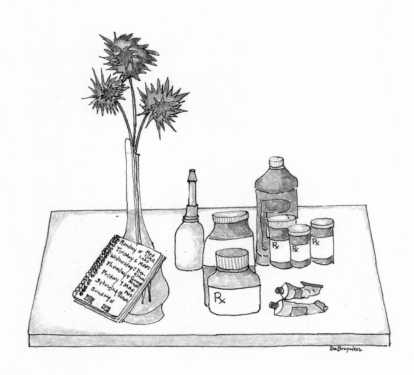

# Being HIV Asymptomatic and Living with an AIDS Diagnosis

## Living with Being HIV Positive

I VISITED WITH JOHN AND CINDY at their duplex on the East Side of St. Paul. Their home looks like any other in the neighborhood—full of the usual clutter associated with a young child in the house. Cindy and her daughter Julie have both tested positive for HIV.

I hadn't visited with Cindy for awhile and I wanted to see how she was doing. She and her daughter have no symptoms at this time, but the emotional stress of living with the virus is a constant presence.

"I'm happy when no one knows I'm positive. I want freedom and privacy and confidentiality. It's hard enough for me that I have to admit to myself that my life could suddenly change—without having people's prejudice change it for me. Even the way people who are here to help treat me is upsetting. I want to be treated normally, not like a piece of china or a time bomb. I'm caught between wanting to be left alone and wanting constant support. If it wasn't for the support group, I think I would be crazy. At least with them I can check out my feelings. I really feel sorry for John. He's caught in the middle.

John reacted to this comment with a kind of helpless shrug of his shoulders. "I'm still on the outside. I can't get inside her head. I can't feel what she feels. I go to the doctor with them, but I can't decide what to do—we're making decisions from different points of view. AZT is an example. I know she takes it to arrest the virus and maybe it's working and maybe it isn't. I don't know. The cost is incredible and we're barely making it now. I want her to be well. I want everything to be okay. I wish I could wake up and the whole thing would have disappeared, been all a mistake. When I'm at work doing some repetitive job, my mind just keeps drifting back to AIDS. I daydream about the awful things that could come and the life we have been cheated out of.

"I heard someone call AIDS the modern day leprosy, and I think of how people with leprosy were treated in the scriptures. Is that us? If it is, then God is definitely on our side. Persons with AIDS are God's greatest fans right now. I know I'm always talking to him now. I've run away from a lot of things in my life. This is the hardest thing I've ever stood up to. We've learned so much about ourselves since this has happened—the disease, the help that's out there. If only we could trust people. We have to be honest, but we can't always. That hurts. If only people could learn with us and not be afraid."

## Bob's Remembrance

THIS ALL HAPPENED about a month after Mom and my sister brought me back to Minnesota. I felt much better, but I was still weak. Mom started sorting through my boxes. She'd hold up things, and I'd say, "Pitch it!" or "Keep it!" We'd just finished sorting a box of old clothes when she pulled out an old shirt box. She moved across the room and sat next to me on the couch.

"I had Gail put all your photos in this box so that they wouldn't get lost. I know you'll want to look at them," she said as she opened the box and started shuffling through the pictures. She picked up one and looked at it for a minute. It was a picture of my friend Rick and myself. "He certainly is an attractive young man," she said. The cue was hardly subtle, but this was a fishing expedition. We could have played hide-and-seek all afternoon, but instead I picked out a picture of my lover, Cal, and told her, "This is what you're looking for." The photograph, which Cal and I had laughingly called our wedding picture, was taken the afternoon we had signed our power-of-attorney papers. To celebrate the legal recognition of our relationship, we had sat for a professional portrait. We looked so young.

I began to pick out other pictures and explain who, what, when, and where. Mom listened intently. As I reconstructed the last seven years of my life and talked about things which were old hat to me, I suddenly realized that this was all new to her.

I had left home seven years before and had kept in touch only by phoning and by coming home for an occasional holiday. I learned to compartmentalize my life and practiced not telling the family anything about what I did away from them. They knew nothing about my loves, the places I went, or even Cal's death. I had simply metioned that a friend had died. Now Mom wanted to know the story, and I found myself enjoying the telling of it. Suddenly the last seven years became a real part of me again. After we sorted through the box, Mom suggested that we purchase some photograph albums and label my pictures. She then got up and removed a family album from the bookcase next to the fireplace. We paged through photographs of me as a baby and of my baptism and first communion. We looked at our family growing up. Mom needed to integrate what she had just learned about my last seven years with what she had always known.

I started coughing, that maddening convulsing cough. My chest hurt; my temples ached. She grabbed me and held on; we both shook. In a couple of minutes I caught my breath and leaned back in the couch. I was breathing deeply and sweating heavily. Mom wiped my forehead with a tissue. She showed me a picture of her and myself when I was seven or eight and had scarlet fever or some other childhood illness. (I was always sick as a child.) In the photograph, I sat on her lap while she held a washcloth on my forehead. "I wish it was that easy now," I said to her. "Get onto my lap," she said.

I protested that I'd crush her. I'd lost a lot of weight but not that much. She insisted. When I crawled on her lap, I almost fell on the floor but she grabbed me in a bear hug. She put her face close to me, and we both started to laugh. Then she leaned back and I heard laughter turn to sobbing; I joined in.

The next day I saw on the mantelpiece with the other family pictures, Cal's and my wedding picture.

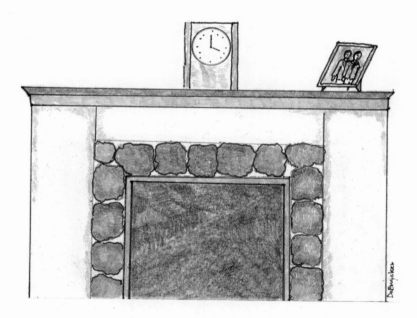

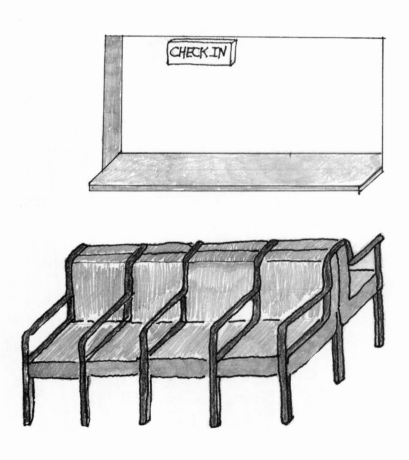

## Jackie's Story

AT FIRST I WOULD WAKE each day with the thought "I have AIDS." This realization pervaded my whole day. I thought about dying, about lost opportunities. I fashioned scenarios of pleasant things I used to do. AIDS destroyed each scene. I imagined myself on a date. I would be dining in a romantic restaurant. At the end of the meal, I'd lean toward my date and whisper, "I have AIDS."

You can imagine the rest. I thought of not seeing my children grow up; I agonized over letting other people raise my children. When I began spending the entire day in bed, dwelling on what might have been, I knew that I'd bottomed out. Then I decided that I had to do something. I thought of suicide but opted instead for a support group. The members of the group cared, but they wouldn't let me wallow in self-pity. They said they couldn't afford to waste time by recounting all their tragedies. They helped me set limited goals for myself—goals I could accomplish in a couple of days or in a few weeks. They also showed me how many decisions I still have control over. They helped me realize that I can make of my life what I want within the limitations of AIDS. The group taught me to celebrate life again.

Actually, in some ways, I have more control over my life now than I did before AIDS. I used to think that I was going to accomplish wonderful things in the future even though I really never planned how these things were to come about. I suffered from feelings of unaccomplishment. Now, I look at things more realistically. I ask myself, "What do I want? Do I have the means to achieve what I'm hoping for? Is it healthy for me? Is it worth the extra risk to accomplish it? Will having it make me happy?"

I'm actually quite amazed at how much I've accomplished. I feel better; my stress level is down; I enjoy people again. I realize that, in the beginning, AIDS accentuated a self-defeating attitude I had about myself. I thought that I was incompetent, that I was no good. Now I no longer envision myself with shame but see myself as a strong person, a person worth knowing.

I hate AIDS, but it's taught me a lot. I wish I would have realized my own worth earlier. No, I actually don't wish this for wishing depresses me. I'll simply stress the positive in my life and let the rest happen. I still wake up in the morning and know that I have AIDS. But now I have too much to accomplish to let this illness keep me in bed. I think I'm beginning to learn how to live one day at a time.

If you have tested HIV positive or have been diagnosed with AIDS:

- Be honest. AIDS provides enough baggage; you don't need the added load of living a lie—neither do those you cherish.

- Rejoice in the aliveness you feel today. Today you're alive! Today is all that anyone can cherish.

- Accept your feelings of grief, but do not let these feelings consume you. Because you may not be able to fulfill your hopes and dreams, you may grieve deeply. But try not to let AIDS become the center of your life.

- Realize that those close to you are also experiencing the loss of dreams and hope. They, too, feel grief— grief for themselves and for you.

- Release yourself from the burden of long-range goals. Project yourself toward the fulfilling of shorter term accomplishments. Revel in the surprise of each new achievement.

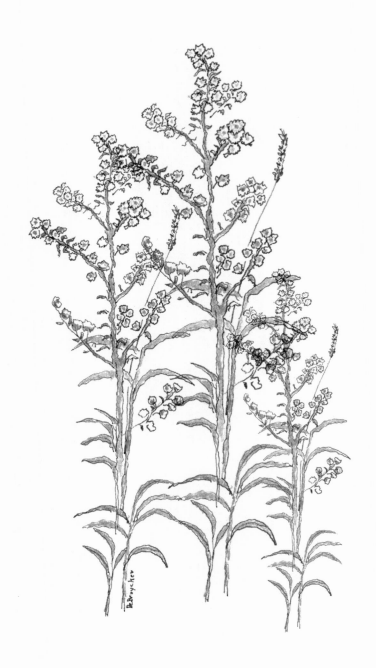

# Families and Friends

## A Parent's Thoughts

THE MORNING WAS beautiful, peaceful. I was wide awake despite having not slept for three days. My only child had been diagnosed with AIDS and given three days to three months to live. I had spent the past three days at his side—first at home, then in the emergency room, and finally at the hospital. I'd spent the days comforting both him and myself. I had a feeling of relief during this time: at least now I knew the reason for his illnesses of the past year and a half. Yet everything—the beauty of the morning and the realization of the prognostication—still seemed unreal.

Questions haunted my waking moments: Whom do I need to tell? What can I say? How do we deal with this? What has to be done? What can we do? Where do I get help, money, service? How do I provide his care? How do I assure my safety? I found myself praying over and over, "Dear God, you are my help in every need!" Then I forced myself to stop this ceaseless round of questioning. I tried to relax and sort out what I really knew from what I could only speculate on. I willed myself to take one step at a time because I knew that I couldn't solve everything at once.

I sipped my coffee and affirmed in prayer my love for my child lying in the hospital bed fighting for his life. With God's help I would have the strength, courage, and fortitude to help him fight for his life regardless of what this fight required of me.

Of one thing I was certain: I could only be available to help him if I took care of myself. I had to tell certain people that he had AIDS because I needed their support, as did he, through prayer and physical help. I began to list questions about places and people to contact for answers. I made a list of people to call and noted what I would say.

Together, my son and I survived the first illness, the second, and several more. This was a time to fight. And, although this was foreign territory, I found that when my son's life was on the line, I could stand firm for what I knew intuitively was right. This was also a time to talk, to love, to relax, to accept that life moves at its own pace. But no time came when we could shut out the reality that AIDS is a deadly illness with no known cure.

As the days passed into months, the illness took its toll on our strength. Anger erupted, but we didn't let it fester. Disappointments came, but they did not become defeats. We changed our goals and accepted each day as a blessing. We made the most of each encounter, and we accepted each new problem as an experience to be worked through. Thus, our days were as good as we could make them. We took advantage of the time we had. We said what we wanted and needed to say. We expressed our love and care for one another and for others. We believed in miracles but lived in the now. We learned that now is all that each of us can be certain about. We rejoiced in our discovery that each hour is wonderful when we love someone and care about one another.

We knew that when the future came we could be content knowing we had been provided the wisdom and the ability to meet each challenge that life presented.

The time came when I could truly say, "It's okay, Honey. Relax, let go; God is with you and with me. Rest in peace—there is no more pain, no more fighting."

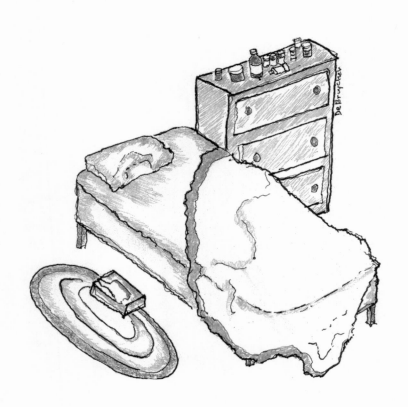

# A Father's Remembrance

I WAITED IN THE HOSPITAL ROOM, with its acrid smell of urine and feces, and listened to the sounds that had become so familiar: the ticking of the intravenous pump; the labored breathing of my son, Josh; and the whistling sound of the air vent above.

The nurse caught my attention as she snapped on her latex gloves. I didn't like this nurse—she always smiled and she always called Josh "cute." "Isn't he the cutest thing!" "Oh, isn't he cute!" Cute was an adjective for dogs or stuffed animals, not for a twenty-five-year-old man. The word said nothing about what my son was enduring with so much perseverance.

She came into the room, fiddled with the bag of intravenous mixture on the pole, reset the pump, and then pulled the needle from the IV on my son's arm. Before leaving, she looked at me and said, "Isn't he a darling!" Only she could have come up with a word that was more grating than cute. Five years before I'd learned that Josh was gay. He'd invited me and my wife, Lois, out for dinner and told us. Josh knew how I hated to go out to those posh quiet little theme restaurants. I had to be quiet, on my best behavior. I'd felt as trapped in that restaurant as I did in the hospital room. But the kid was smart—he knew that inviting me out to eat was probably the only way he could get me to listen for a whole hour.

With no introduction, Josh blurted out his gayness between dinner and dessert. We met his statement with dead silence. Thoughts raced through my mind: Was I angry? How did I really feel? Did Josh expect me to be Mr. Liberal? Lois responded first. "We love you, Josh. Just as you are."

"Shit" was the only word that came to my mind, but I didn't say it. Instead I said something even worse. "Thank God! I thought you were going to tell me you were a Republican!" Both Josh and Lois looked at me as if I were from outer space. I always tried to joke my way out of everything, but once again I stuck my foot in my mouth. Then I jammed it in even farther by blowing up and snarling, "Well what do you want me to do? Stand up and have everyone give three cheers for my queer son!" I said that loud enough for the people at the nearby tables to hear. I ruined dessert and landed in the doghouse for three months.

I handled the news about Josh's AIDS much better than I did the revelation of his gayness. I'm a natural fixer. I immediately tried to take control: "Are you sure?" "Have you been tested?" "Who's your doctor?" "Is he any good?" "You have to move home right away." "We can fix up the bedroom." Even before I ended my questioning, I realized that I was driving Josh nuts. Lois just held him and cried. I wish I could have done that.

The next months were busy. We kept in constant touch with Josh. I took him to the clinic and kept on him constantly to make sure he was taking his medication. I talked with his doctors and tried to make sure that I knew everything about Josh's condition. I even drew up charts of his T-cell counts, although I hid these in my ledger with my stock charts. I collected a bigger AIDS library than the doctors had. I even started lighting votive candles at church—something I hadn't done for years. But even as I fought to control the disease, I was scared. Soon my greatest fear came to pass, for Josh started losing weight; he was tired and had diarrhea all the time. When he started to have problems breathing, he went into the hospital. I knew it was PCP, the pneumonia that so frequently comes with AIDS.

Lois kept saying, "Why don't you talk to Josh? He needs to know you love him." What did she want from me? I wasn't good at mushy stuff; whenever I tried to tell Josh how much I cared, I'd end up making some stupid joke. "I should have thrown the ball to McDonough." Josh's voice started me from my hospital reverie. He was awake and looking up at the ceiling.

"What are you talking about?" I asked.

"I said I should have thrown the ball to McDonough."

"Who the hell is McDonough?"

"Don't you remember? He was the center on St. Kevin's basketball team in eighth grade. It was the last game of the year, and I got the rebound and instead of passing the ball I tried to take it all the way down court by myself. I fell and lost the game."

"I can't believe you're still upset about that; it was so long ago."

"But I remember it," Josh said. "I knew I'd let you down; you didn't say anything the whole way home. I knew you were angry with me. I tried real hard for you; I wanted you to be proud of me."

"You don't know me very well do you, Josh? That's probably my fault. I wasn't angry at you! I was angry at that ass of a coach. I knew you tried hard; that S.O.B. was so unfair to you and the other boys. He never gave any of you any credit. I could never understand why you worked so hard." "You never said anything to me, Dad." Tears filled Josh's eyes.

I could feel myself lose control. My mind started racing for an escape clause. I couldn't find any. To hell with McDonough. I did something I'd never done before. I grabbed Josh in my arms and shook with tears.

# Coming Home

I N NOVEMBER, WHEN I RETURNED to work from my maternity leave, Paul was one of the first patients I met. He had been on Hospice Service since the summer before. Both Johnna Edmunds and Suzanne Chevalier were seeing him, Johnna as his hospice nurse and Suzanne as his volunteer.

Paul had been affected early in life by a moderately disabling disease. Nonetheless, he had grown up and was living on his own as a young adult when he became ill. He was diagnosed with a terminal disease. It was then that he returned home. The effect of one disease process in combination with another took its toll on Paul. By the time I met him, he was confined to bed. He spent virtually all of his time on his back, unable to turn or be comfortable unless fairly flat in bed. He had only limited use of his arms and legs.

Paul's mother, Mary, was wonderfully supportive. Sometimes I thought that she breathed the very life into Paul, their home, and their world. Her home was always warm and inviting. It was common to find two or more women cheerfully working away in the kitchen, "egging" as they called it. You see, Mary is an artist and teacher in the hobby of creating beautiful ornaments and keepsakes from eggs of all sizes and sorts. At Christmas, she decorated a special miniature tree for Paul. It was all done up with the most delightful ornaments—all eggs! And even though

Paul didn't make much of a fuss about it, I knew that he was very proud of his mother, her talent, and her devotion to him. Just as Mary was an artist with her eggs, so she was also in her caring for Paul. She was a master at preventing problems and in treating the ones that just could not be prevented. She was Paul's dietician, physical therapist, nurse, skin care specialist, and masseuse. She taught me techniques in skin care and the prevention of decubitus ulcer formation that I hope to be able to share with others.

Mary was a woman with a purpose. Her mission was to care for Paul and to keep him home for the duration. She approached each day with thoughtful determination. I know that God and her faith in him were powerful forces supporting her and guiding her day by day as she cared for Paul. She told me after Paul's death that taking care of Paul was a privilege. I hadn't exactly realized it, but that is how I felt—privileged—as I entered their home to be a part of their loving plan.

Paul had been described as quiet and withdrawn. True enough, he was quiet by nature, but friendly and thought-ful. He didn't talk about himself a great deal. He seemed more interested in others, you know, in the small details that make up our own lives. He seemed quite serene and accepting of his eventual death. And he also seemed very well adjusted to his limited and often painful physical state as a mostly acceptable way to live. Each time I visited, I felt a growing appreciation for how Paul and Mary lived each day with grace and dignity.

As Paul's condition deteriorated, his physical care needs became overwhelming at times, even for Mary. She did receive help and support from her daughters, Paul's doctor, their friends, paid nursing, and Hospice staff and volunteers, but her own physical problems flared up under the stress and grief she experienced, rendering her almost unable to walk. Then help came in the form of Sister Nan. Nan, a nun and Mary's sibling, was truly a gift from God. She came by plane, but may as well have descended directly from heaven! With such great energy, honesty, humor and sense of purpose, Nan supported Mary as no other human could. She cared for Mary and she cared for Paul when Mary could not. But in testimony to Mary's flawless care and Paul's reluctance to let go of this world as his body failed, she exclaimed, "Now why would Paul want to die? He already has heaven right here on earth!"

And Mary and Nan succeeded in keeping Paul home. He was able to die as he had lived, surrounded by family loving him to the end of this life—and wishing him well for the life that awaited him on the other side.

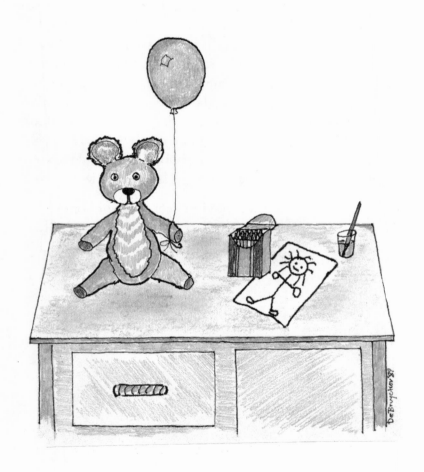

## Talking to Children about AIDS

WHEN TALKING TO young children about AIDS or any life-threatening situation, it is important to remember that children are self-referent. This means that they interpret the world as if all events that take place occur because of them, because of how they have behaved, or because they have wished for something.

Children need to be reassured that AIDS, divorce and unemployment are not their fault and not under their control. They can be reassured that AIDS can't be caught easily and that the adults in their life can and will protect them from AIDS.

Along the same lines, children are dependent on adults. That their dependence is physical, emotional and financial is obvious even to them. If you are the parent or guardian of a child, you need to remind the child that he/she will be taken care of if you should become ill or die. If you are HIV infected, your child needs to know who will take care of him/her if you become too ill to do so, and what long term plans you've made for his/her care. If you are not HIV infected, it would still be wise to reassure your child that you have contingency plans for his or her care, since all children have fears of abandonment when they are old enough to understand that their parents and caregivers are mortal.

At five, my son Sam was afraid his daddy and I would get AIDS and no one would take care of him. When we explained that we had a will and what that meant to him, he bounced happily out to play with no more questions. On the other hand, my eight-year-old daughter Hilary was very frightened by the information she'd been given at school. She was particularly upset at being told that you can have AIDS and not know it. Unfortunately, the school hadn't told her how the virus is transmitted, leaving her to her fears with inadequate information. She needed reassurance that she was all right and information on how the virus spread before she was calm enough to ask me if I had AIDS and what would happen if I became ill.

I believe that children need to have all their questions about AIDS answered. Very young children will ask simpler and less technical questions and their fears will be very direct, i.e., Will you die? When? Who will love me if you die?

An older child needs to be reassured that he or she will be cared for and given specific information about the disease. It does no one any good to be told about AIDS' existence and then denied the facts necessary to understand and make choices to protect themselves. As the parent of a boy and a girl, I have had to answer questions that were intimate and at times uncomfortable, but the discomfort was far outweighed by the trust my children have given me— and also by the growth in my own understanding of AIDS and my beliefs about life.

Finally, deeds speak louder than words. We don't just talk about the hungry, we give money and food to the food banks. We don't just say we are in favor of the truth, we tell the truth.

My children were glad to have me answer their questions, but their fears were truly laid to rest when they saw me eat dinner with a friend who has AIDS. Bill and I have been friends since high school. News of his illness made me cry, and my kids were sad because I was sad. They had a lot of questions for Bill, some funny and some poignant. Both of my children know that AIDS doesn't have to kill love or friendship—and that has proven the best education of all.

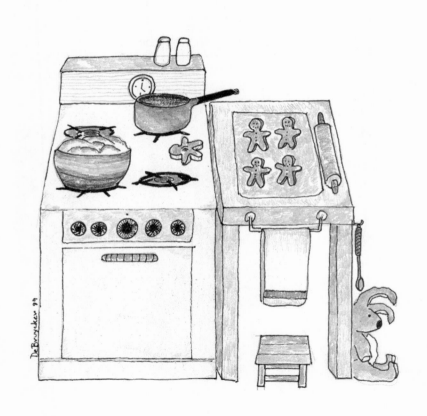

## Keith and Alex

THERE ARE SEVERAL important children in my life these days. Most are nieces and nephews. One is my friend Alex who is three years old. In my previous years as a social worker with children and their families and with my studies in early childhood development, I learned a lot about talking with children. Since being diagnosed with AIDS, I've learned a lot more.

There are currently many resources to assist families in prevention education. What I will be discussing is how to talk to children when someone they love or who is important in their life is diagnosed.

Most of my family lives in Iowa, 400 miles away. I don't see them often, but I remain connected and involved. I particularly cherish what time I have with my nieces and nephews, who range in age from infants to adults. Since my diagnosis, I have attempted to visit a bit more frequently. I realized fairly early on that my family, though supportive, was not going to deal with this at the pace and in the manner that I would have chosen. I accepted they would follow their own process, and I would participate as much as I could while respecting my own needs.

For the first year and a half, AIDS, and the fact that I have AIDS, was not discussed openly in family situations. There were many conversations one to one with my mother and some with individual siblings. Some of my siblings have still not talked with me directly about AIDS.

Last Thanksgiving, when I went to my parents' home, my mother asked me to bring a copy of *The Quilt, Stories from the Names Project*. A sister had asked for it for Christmas and my mother was unable to find it.

After a very crowded dinner for 32 in my parents' two bedroom home, the tables were cleared and many of us were hanging out in the dining room chatting, eating pie, and laughing.

The sister, Sharon, for whom I bought the book, was unable to be there. My mother asked if I brought the book and suggested that I bring it out for another sister, Rita, to look at. The book includes part of my story, and my mother's suggestion to bring it out felt like an invitation to begin more open discussion. I decided to use this opportunity and also brought out a copy of *Equal Time* in which there was a feature article about me. *The Color of Light* just happened to be in my suitcase, too. What I hoped to accomplish was the sharing of some of what my life is about in a situation where there is not much context. The books and the article were passed around and there were several questions and comments.

The kids were watching all this and vying for their share of attention. Several of my nieces and a nephew finally asked if they could read the article; eleven-year-old Lisa wanted to read it to the younger children. I told them to ask their parents if it was okay. They took the article and went into the other room.

About three minutes later, six-year-old Randy, a very direct and oftentimes defiant little girl, was back to report.

Randy: "I have some questions."

Me: "Okay. What are they?"

Randy: "What is gay and what is AIDS?"

I have a reputation in my family as being "nontraditional" and possibly even eccentric. My ideas on raising children are especially suspect. The adults around the table exchanged those "what now?" looks.

Me: "Well, most people have primary (oh, no, meaningless word for the age level) or important relationships with the opposite sex. If you're a gay man, though, your important relationships are with other men. If you're a gay woman, your important relationships are with other women. (More sidelong glances.)

"AIDS is a disease that affects your immune system. Most people have an immune system that is strong and keeps them from getting sick most of the time. When a person has AIDS, their immune system doesn't work and they get sick with other diseases that most people never get."

Randy: "Do you have AIDS?"

Me: "Yes." (pause) "Do you have questions about that?" (pause)

Randy: "How do you get AIDS?"

Me: "First of all, you don't need to worry about getting AIDS from me. Nothing that you and I would ever do together would give you AIDS. You won't get AIDS by hugging me or drinking out of my cup. You can only get AIDS by being sexual with someone who has it or by shooting drugs with needles that someone else has already used."

Randy: "How did you get it?"

Me: "I was sexual with someone who had it."

Randy: "Well, what girl gave it to you?"

(At this point, several adults chuckled and I realized we had gone about as far as we could with this conversation.)

Me: "I don't know who gave it to me, hon. That isn't too important. You'll probably have some more questions later. It's okay to ask them."

(She turned her attention to the article and read aloud with first grade skill, several times, the opening paragraph, "Keith Gann, a gay man with AIDS...," apparently experimenting with what it sounded and felt like.)

One of the really interesting things about this exchange was that Randy's directness and my candidness suddenly gave adults permission to discuss it. I had several important conversations with adult members of my family as a result of my talk with her.

Alex and I became friends after my diagnosis. One afternoon in August, a year and a half ago, his mother Ann called. She is a member of my Quaker meeting. I knew who she was, but had not really had much contact with her or Alex. She said Alex's father was not involved with him, and she wanted him to grow up knowing there were men in his life who loved and cared about him. She had asked around the meeting and several people had mentioned me as someone who is good with kids. Would I be his friend?

I said yes, but I wasn't certain if she knew I was diagnosed and she needed to in order to be responsible for Alex's well-being and also that there was the possibility that he might have to deal with the loss of me at some point. She responded: "Well, I didn't know that, but everything I've read says Alex would be in no danger of catching AIDS from you. If we have to deal with loss, we'll do it when it happens. Meanwhile, how about it?" I said yes, and Alex and I have spent time together on about a weekly basis ever since. He has been a real joy in my life.

Though I had made some assumptions that Ann was fairly open with him on most issues, including sexuality, I was uncertain what to say when about a year ago he discovered some "gold coin" condoms on my desk and was convinced they were chocolates and I was holding out on him. When Ann picked him up, I explained what had happened and asked her how she would like me to handle future questions about sex or AIDS. She essentially said she trusted my judgment and that the topics were definitely open for discussion.

Several weeks later, he was at my house baking cookies. I suddenly had some dizziness and had to lie down for a minute. He came and sat on the bed, snuggling as close as he could.

"Do you have a disease?"

"Yes."

"What is it?"

"AIDS. Do you know what that is?"

"No."

"Well, it's when your body isn't working quite right and you can't fight off diseases that most people can fight off."

"Will you die?"

"Eventually, everybody dies, one way or another. I don't know if I will die of AIDS or not."

During the next several weeks, he continued to ask questions, sometimes by surprise and always direct, often-times about death and dying. Ann and I both respond to the questions simply and honestly, and as well as we can. Sometimes it feels right and sometimes it feels inadequate. It is always a learning experience for all of us.

Me: "I'm going to a memorial service."

Alex: "What's that?"

Me: "A friend died from AIDS and his friends are getting together to remember him."

Alex: "Why did he die before you?"

Me: "Well, that's a question I don't know the answer to."

I had my second annual survival party and Jello Mold Competition last month. It was important, Ann and I decided, that Alex could come and help celebrate my life with me. He did and had a great time.

We were driving with a friend one day and Alex suddenly said, "Someone in this car might die." Doug, my friend, thought he was thinking about a car accident and said something to the effect that we'll drive carefully. He said, "No, Keith might die of a disease."

Me: "Well, yes, that's possible, but I don't really have any plans to do that right away."

Alex: "Kids don't die."

Me: "Not usually, but sometimes. No one really knows when someone will die."

Alex: "Well, you can't die. You have to get a lot older first."

I smiled. I wish I had said, "Oh, Alex, I sure love you and I hope you're right. I would really like to be with you as you grow up. I can't say for certain that I will be. But I'm doing all the important things to make life happy, and maybe long, like laughing, and dancing, and eating, and sleeping, and loving, and playing. For however long it lasts. I'm glad that you and I are doing it together!"

There will undoubtedly be another opportunity…he tends to push a point.

**Tips:**

Though I don't claim the definitive understanding of talking to kids about AIDS, here are a few hints I've found helpful.

1.  If the child is not yours, try to have an understanding beforehand of the parents' values and attitudes about such discussions.

2.  Be simple and direct. The child will ask as many questions as needed.

3.  Be honest.

4.  It's okay to say, "I don't know the answer to that one."

5.  Reassure the child that she/he is not in danger of getting AIDS.

6.  Give lots of permission to ask questions.

7.  Children, particularly young children, do not always process information sequentially. Questions and comments will come up in unexpected places and at unexpected times. Respond to them as they arise.

8.  Children may need to go through things several times and may repeat the same question or catch phrases as

they build a framework into which to fit the information.

9. Tell the child where to go to ask more questions, i.e., yourself, a parent, a trusted teacher, other family members.

10. You don't have to do it perfectly.

11. Love yourself and love the child. Tell them!

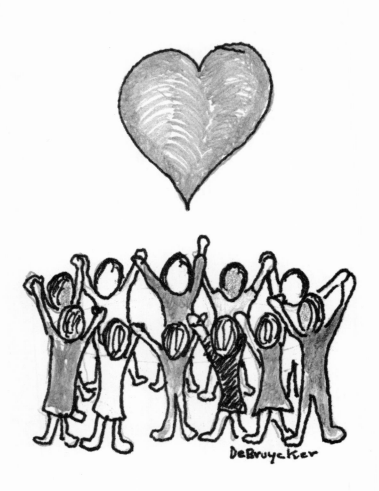

# Care Givers

*The author of this introduction is a senior social worker at a major Midwestern hospital.*

A DIAGNOSIS OF HIV+ OR AIDS is wrought with psychosocial issues, concerns and potential conflict. Need for information and resource coordination, to accompany competent medical assessment and management alternatives, is immediate and frequently overwhelming for those touched by this diagnosis.

We who are support people have opportunity to bring non-judgmental information and unconditional caring to those in need of both. We can offer to people living with a diagnosis of HIV+/ARC/AIDS the trust and peace inherent in a caregiver's competent presence.

The following points are offered from my perspective for the initial direction of volunteers, caregivers and support people:

Be aware of the diagnosis a person is dealing with: HIV+? ARC? AIDS? How does the individual perceive the diagnosis intellectually and emotionally?

Be aware of the individual's risk behavior which enabled transmission to support, when appropriate, movement toward altering that behavior to maximize future health.

Inquire about and seek to understand the environment the patient comes from including education, employment, lifestyle, and use of mood-altering chemicals.

Seek information regarding past experiences coping with stress to identify strengths to draw upon as positive coping mechanisms.

Who is in the individual's support system? Has he/she shared the HIV+ or AIDS diagnosis with a family member or friend? If there is no support, how might he/she choose to incorporate an available support person or group into his/her lifestyle?

Medical social workers and/or case management professionals generally have responsibility for offering informed financial direction regarding healthcare alternatives in the treatment of HIV+/AIDS and are appropriate resources for financial concerns. Planning proactive medical management of the disease process includes anticipating financial concerns to minimize accompanying stress.

# Suggestions for Care Givers

*The author has been living with the spectre of AIDS for almost two years. A social activist, he remains committed and involved in education for justice.*

WHEN I WAS diagnosed with AIDS Related Complex (ARC) in February of 1988, I was emotionally, physically, and spiritually devastated. My world had exploded into a wasteland that projected only isolation, fear, and hopelessness. To protect myself, I went into a personal exile.

Gradually I emerged from this darkness and experienced those patented stages identified with having a life-threatening illness: anger, denial, grief, bargaining, and eventually acceptance. I still continue to struggle physically, emotionally, and spiritually with this disease but with one critical difference: I now accept the care of the people in my life who support me on my journey toward healing and wholeness.

Over the last year I have been blessed with a wonderful team of people who love me and support me through both the good and the bad times. I'd like to share some suggestions from my experience that can perhaps help others as they reach out to those who live with AIDS.

- Ask about the illness, but be sensitive to whether your friend wants to discuss it.

- Learn how to be comfortable with silence. Sitting together and reading, listening to music, watching television, or holding hands is a good means of support and comfort. Much can be expressed without words.

- Encourage your friend to make decisions. Living with AIDS can cause a loss of control over many aspects of life. Don't deny your friend a chance to make decisions, no matter how simple or silly these decisions may seem to you.

- Be prepared for your friend to get angry with you even if you've done everything you could for him or her. Remember that anger is often taken out on the people closest because they are safe and will understand and forgive.

- Keep your friend up to date on the latest news. Talk about your common interests. Your friend may be tired of talking about symptoms, doctors, and treatments. Small talk can be healthy.

- Go for a walk or outing together, but ask about and know your friend's endurance limitations.

- Touch your friend. A simple squeeze of the hand or a hug can let her or him know that you care. Hugs are very reassuring.

- Call before coming to visit. If your friend is tired that day, visit on another occasion. By your support and care, help your friend keep loneliness and fear at a distance. But try to be supportive of your friend when he or she can not keep loneliness and fear at bay.

- Do not confuse acceptance of the illness with defeat. By accepting the illness your friend may experience a sense of his or her own power.

- Beware of lecturing your friend if she or he seems to be handling the illness in a way that you think is inappropriate. Your friend may not be where you expect or need him or her to be. You may not understand what the feelings are and why certain choices are being made.

- If you and your friend are religious, ask if you could pray together. Don't be hesitant to share your faith. Spirituality can be critical at this time.

- Be realistic with your friend. If he or she looks good, say so but do not lie. If your friend's appearance has changed, respond to this change. Be gentle.

- Use your creativity. Bring books, periodicals, puzzles, taped music, home-baked cookies, or photographs to share. All of these simple things can bring warmth and joy into your friend's life.

- Help keep your friend part of a group; don't allow your friend or his or her significant other to become isolated. Talk about support groups and other services that are offered without charge.

- Be positive, for this attitude is catching.

- Talk with your friend about the future: tomorrow, next week, next year. Looking forward to the future without denying the reality of today is always good. Hope is critical at this time.

- Offer to help answer any correspondence which may be giving some difficulty or which your friend is avoiding.

- Offer to do household chores. You might do the laundry, wash dishes, water plants, buy groceries. This may be appreciated more than you realize. However, don't do what your friend wants to do and can still do for herself or himself. Ask before doing anything.

- Finally, take care of yourself! Recognize your own emotions and honor them. Share your grief and anger, your feelings of helplessness with your own support group. Getting the support you need during this crisis will help you to be the real friend for your friend.

# Being a Care Giver

*The author, a gay man, has been an AIDS volunteer and
minister for four years.*

BEING A VOLUNTEER who ministers to people
living with AIDS is a privilege. In the course of
the disease, people living with AIDS and their
extended families may grieve many losses: health,
financial stability, career, long-range dreams. They feel and
express strong emotions, including guilt, fear, and anger.
One of the ways I can help is to be a nonjudgmental and
supportive friend at these times. Sometimes those touched
by AIDS can't find the words to share their hurt; they
simply want someone to be with them. Just being present
is difficult for a "do-gooder" like myself. I'd like to fix
things and provide the right answers to make everything
better. But people living with AIDS need to have control
over as much of their lives as possible. Feeling overwhelmed
by the uncontrollable aspects of the disease, they need to
experience the power of making decisions related to their
treatment, comfort, and environment.

From my work as a volunteer, I've gained appreciation for
and sensitivity to the highs and lows of life. I've learned to
live in the present. I've learned the immeasurable values of
small things shared—a laugh, a cry, a silent moment or a
hug. These intangible gifts are precious.

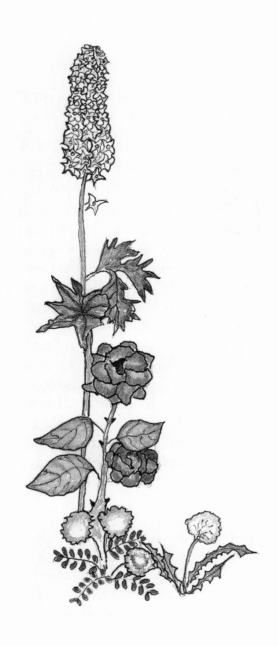

## Being a Volunteer

AT THE CONCLUSION of a seminar on AIDS at the College of Saint Thomas, a request was made for volunteers. I thought, "Why not volunteer? I'm retired; I have time; I know members of the gay community, people who might be affected by AIDS; there's a need." So, I volunteered.

In any service, you always receive more in return than you give. (My Irish father would say, "God will never be outdone in generosity.")

What have I received from the AIDS ministry? Mine has been a faith experience. The ministry has changed what was, for me, simply "faith" to a "living faith." I have encountered Christ in being a driver, while holding a hand, while helping plan a fund raiser. Christ is in all acts of service and in all expressions of compassion and love. The same encounters have given me the opportunity to be open to new loves and new friends who both confirm and encourage me. My reward has been learning that Christ is encountered in the midst of daily living.

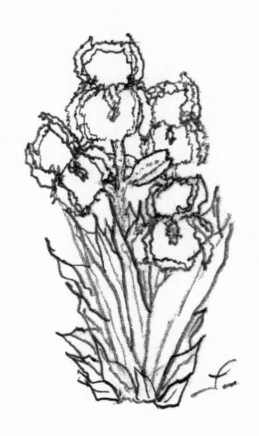

## The Rewards of Volunteering

WHEN I BEGAN my experience as a volunteer, I was filled with fear, anxiety, and myriad questions: How would I talk to this stranger? What if we didn't like each other? What could I possibly do to help him?

During the months that have followed, Jim and I have become good friends. He is important to me, and I look forward to our weekly visits. Jim has been very open in letting me know what he needs and how I can best help him.

I remained amazed by his courage—courage to fight this disease and courage to accept it. I am inspired by his appreciation for each day, and I find I have a greater awareness of how precious this gift of life is. I am saddened at how fragile he is—how vulnerable.

I am much more aware of the goodness in others as I observe the many kindnesses people extend to him: mowing his lawn, doing his laundry, shopping for groceries, cooking for him, bringing fresh flowers. Watching how much joy these simple acts provide brings me a great deal of pleasure.

Jim has given me and all his friends the opportunity to experience the gift of sharing ourselves, not only with him but with one another. So many people come together because of Jim.

Spending this time with Jim has forced me to accept pain and suffering and unfinished goals as a part of life. But this time has also made me aware that God is present in all life experiences.

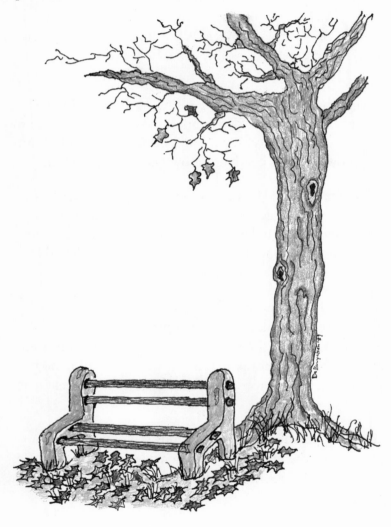

# Grieving

URING YOUR LIFETIME you have experienced both loss and grief. Each time a hope, dream, or actual expectation didn't materialize, you lost a bit of your self, a bit of your energy for the moment and for the future.

Grief makes you vulnerable to fatigue, error, illness, and loss of concentration. While grieving, the task you would have completed in an hour takes days. You can't make the simplest of decisions because you are unable to focus on the problems you face. You are unable to finish the book you once could have read in an evening. Moreover, forcing yourself to accomplish your daily tasks takes energy you don't have at this time. Forcing an issue results in error and decisions that you will regret later.

Accept these facts about your grief. Be kind to yourself. Say "No" to demands; if you've already said "Yes," admit your inability to handle the situation at this time. The author of Ecclesiastes says that a time comes to give and to receive, to sow and to reap. Let this be your time of healing—healing for your body, your mind, and your soul.

During this time of healing, your concentration will return. Then you can deal with new demands, then you can make plans, then you can again dream dreams, then you can hope and look to new horizons.

Be assured that everyone grieves differently. You need to take time to grieve—this is essential for you. In fact, the more you feel the pain, the sooner you can get through it and resolve it. You will know that your grief is resolved when you can remember your loved one without pain or grief. Then the good memories will return.

Remember that the process of grieving is personal to you. You do not need to fit someone else's time schedule. You do, however, need to take care of yourself. Be kind and gentle to yourself, but try to avoid letting the feelings of helplessness prevent you from getting on with your daily life. Acknowledge your feelings of helplessness, anger, guilt, and denial, but then let go of these feelings and let good memories flood your heart.

Let grief run its course. Experience the anger, the pain, the sadness, the loss of concentration and energy. Hurting is okay. You have a reason to hurt.

When the mending begins, pick up the small sticks of your life one at a time. Eventually you will again have the will and the strength to lift the whole bundle.

# A Mother Reflects on Grieving

AIDS HAS TAKEN FROM ME the son I loved, and continue to love, more dearly than life. If your experience is like mine, it will initiate a spiritual crisis unlike anything you have ever known. Do not try to minimize its meaning or its power. God is ever present. Pray, even when all your heart can formulate is an agonized cry of helplessness. Remember the unconditional love with which you embraced your son during his illness. You surrounded him with acceptance and openness. Count the many spiritual gifts your son gave you in his living and in his dying. My son shared with me his love, his courage, his faith, his concern, and his specialness. Now that he is dead, I treasure these gifts more than gold.

Christ's love has come to me through the caring and compassion I have received from others. Right now, in your grief, you need and deserve support. Seek and accept the company and comfort of others whom you feel are helpful to you. But trust yourself on what you are ready to deal with and do not let any externally imposed guidelines or well-meaning others rush or impede that process. We do not "get over" our grief; it is a process that we must walk through.

As you grieve, be open to the whole gamut of emotions. They are all acceptable and necessary and they do not need to be judged. Try, try, and keep on trying, especially when you feel like succumbing to hopelessness. Confront your fears because fear and compassion are incompatible. During this time of grief, do not expect too much of yourself. Regressing is okay, and you will probably find yourself going back over the same memories and regrets and feelings again and again. But try to practice letting go. When you are willing to let your experience and love create a future, new meaning will come to your life. Let your sorely wounded spirit be open to growth in grace. Resolve to honor your son by continuing to live and love with purpose and meaning. My son asked that of me and I am sure your son would want it of you.

## How to Help Someone Who Is Grieving

The Compassionate Friend, an organization of support groups for the bereaved, suggests that people can best help bereaved friends by remembering the "Five B's."

1. Be there.

2. Be quiet.

3. Be attentive. (Don't make decisions for the bereaved but give them choices—about the funeral, what to do with the deceased's clothing, and so on.)

4. Be patient. (A long time passes before the intense feelings subside. In the meantime, the bereaved need to talk about the death.)

5. Be remembering. (Remember the deceased at holidays; mention her or his positive, enduring traits. Don't

worry that you will be "reminding" the bereaved of something they have forgotten. If anything, you will show your friends that you have not forgotten.)

## Other Advice on Helping the Bereaved

- ❧ Do say you are sorry.

- ❧ Encourage the bereaved to express as much grief as they want.

- ❧ Forget your own sense of discomfort and reach out to the bereaved.

- ❧ Be willing to talk about the deceased.

- ❧ Avoid trying to find something positive to say about the deceased's death. Don't point out to the bereaved that at least they have other children, friends, family, and so on.

- ❧ Avoid making comments suggesting that medical care given to the deceased was inadequate, and so on.

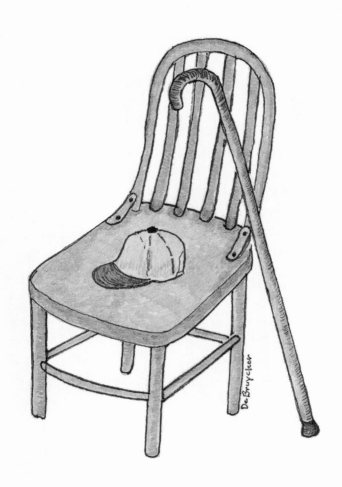

## Empowering Journey

*The following excerpt is from an article by a young man who was his spouse's main caregiver until his spouse died from AIDS. He gives us insights into the issues that surround caring for a person with AIDS (PWA), highlighting the emotional roller-coaster an AIDS diagnosis puts one on and its impact on feelings, attitudes and relationships.*

DEALING WITH AIDS has changed my life completely. I would like to talk about some different aspects of my experience.

It is very hard for individuals to deal with a chronic illness. The weakness, the losses and the grieving bring one's own mortality into perspective. Confronted with this situation, individuals find it much easier not to deal with it and to pretend nothing has changed. It is human nature to pretend one can make something go away if one ignores it.

At the beginning of my lover's and my ordeal, people seemed to be very attentive to our needs. They seemed well intentioned towards helping, often saying, "Please call if you need help." I quickly realized that this response was easier for people to say than it was to act on. It was easier to deal with people who said, "I have two or three hours to spare," or "I will bring you dinner," or "I will come and clean your windows or mow the lawn for you."

This brings me to the heart of caregiving. No matter if you are the primary caregiver, a family member or friend, you are the one who must choose to do it, to make a decision to give care. I insist on the word "decide" because we all have choices and decisions to make in life. (I remember my spouse once asking me to decide between being with him in his illness to help him, or leaving him if I needed to.) This is the first step one must take in order to joyfully accept the challenges of caring for another person and adapting to new and difficult situations brought about by everyday changes.

I remember once going away for some "me-time" to re-examine and re-evaluate my own commitment to my spouse. Before leaving, I took out our personal directory and drew up a list of names of people I could count on for help. This was a very revealing experience. I sensed myself feeling left out by so many. For my own health, I came to realize that I had to learn how to ask for a commitment from others, how to invite them into service, and how to ask for help.

This brings me to the second great principle of caregiving: if you have made the decision and commitment to care for another person, then you must care also for yourself. You are not God; you cannot do everything—and you can do even less if you are exhausted. So take care of yourself, let others help you, ask for the help, and take time off.

No matter how great the commitment you make to help, the constant and sometimes rapid changes in the health, finances, attitudes and feelings of a chronically ill person put stress on the caregiver. The changes challenge and redefine one's relationships, attitudes, and communication with the PWA and others, as well as one's own feelings. (Feelings are often left aside because of our fear of dealing with deep emotions.)

AIDS brings alterations to a relationship, but basically the relationship continues in the same manner as before the illness. It is therefore important to try to understand what had been going on in the relationship before the diagnosis and how that will affect the caregiver's role. This includes all relationships—with oneself, significant other, family and friends. One should keep in mind that the specter of death and issues around sexuality are such intimate aspects of our lives that, even without the stress of illness, they can be expected to impact our relationship.

Another impact on our relationships as well as on any given life situation is our attitude. People can be optimistic, pessimistic or realistic to various degrees about every aspect of life. It is important to know the PWA's attitude towards life as well as your own. (Once again, this will probably be the same as before the illness.) This knowledge allows you to understand each other's needs and complement each other and helps you know when you need some outside support or guidance.

The PWA may hold a variety of attitudes toward his or her illness, which may change over the course of the illness. The PWA may be the "wounded lion" who likes to be left alone and is not very appreciative of your help. Or the PWA may be the "happy warrior" who needs a crowd of people around and is very supportive and appreciative of your help. Sometimes the PWA switches back and forth between both attitudes, which can be very confusing and painful to you.

The attitudes of others should also be recognized and some-times even defended against. These attitudes can affect the health and well-being of the PWA and his or her caregivers, family and friends. Often you can feel the sub-tle—or sometimes not so subtle—pressure from family and friends saying, "You have a terminal or chronic illness, you should be morose, you should quit celebrating, you should hurry up and die." (Of course, the greater the fear of death and intimacy, the more acute the attitude.) My lover and I had to fight to maintain an attitude of normalcy. Always remember that you are fully alive until the moment you stop breathing. This can give you the energy to live and the ability to mourn and grieve when you have to, not before. Remember, every change implies a loss and there-fore some grieving. There are lots of losses in AIDS, so learn to talk about them, learn to communicate among yourselves and others.

Effective communication comes from active listening, response and participation. It is not easy. Talking about death is not easy. My first conversations with my lover were painful. We are not trained to thing in terms of our own death, especially at a young age. We grew by talking about his eventual death. You can come to grips with wills, funeral arrangements, memorial services, and the meaning death has for you and the PWA. You may even develop a stress relieving kind of "black humor" about all these things. You can change your attitude toward death so that it seems less fearful—until, finally, it has meaning and hope. Communication allows you to discuss each treatment, your hopes and fears for the future, and your anger and sadness. It also allows you to identify and celebrate your joy. Without communication it is hard to know what to celebrate and what to grieve. Communication helps you know your own feelings.

Dealing with your feelings and those of the PWA is an emotional roller-coaster ride, often from anger to despair, to sadness, to joy, and back to anger again. You play mind games trying to deal with your grief and keeping on an even keel for the sake of the person you are caring for. You might pretend everything is going well until you are brought suddenly back to reality by a new crisis. You might become paranoid about the medical and social service establishment: "Do they think we are guinea pigs? Why won't they tell us anything without our begging them? Aren't they listening to us? Don't they realize we are only human?" Your feelings may begin to distort your thinking. You'll be taxed and frustrated by the medical bureaucracy, social security, insurance companies and family, all when you feel most powerless and at your lowest ebb of energy. "How do we get to the doctor, the clinic, the pharmacy?" "How can we make house payments, buy groceries, pay for medicine?" "What do you mean, a nursing home?" "Do I have to stay in the hospital?" "Why can't I stay in the hospital?" All of this seems so overwhelming that it becomes very hard to cope. As time goes on, there is so much to do, it's easy to begin to feel that you are responsible for everything and to become resentful. And the more resentful you become, the guiltier you feel. This is the time to go back to the beginning: You have made a decision to care for this person; you are not God; you need to take care of yourself. You are a good person of value who is fighting against overwhelming odds. It's time to call for help.

The role of caregiver, although a difficult one, puts you in touch with the real world. It helps you redefine your life as you re-examine your value system. It lets you know that every day is worth living to its fullest, and that it is in giving of ourselves to others that we grow and learn the meaning of life. I know that I will never be the same.

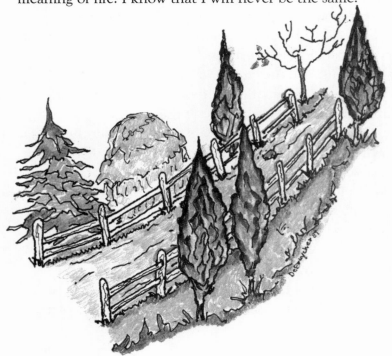

## Thoughts I Share...

I WAS DIAGNOSED HIV-POSITIVE five years ago, in 1986, and had suspected I was infected for a period before this, so I have been dealing with this condition for a long time. In 1985, I had a lymph node biopsy which showed no cancerous infection, but marked the beginning of the medical process. I did quite well for a number of years, even though it was a terrible secret to keep in a time of hysteria about AIDS. I pulled back from people because I didn't want them to know and I didn't want any possibility of infecting anyone. It was a period of fear, shame and isolation.

In March of 1989, I became seriously ill and was hospitalized. At that time I not only had to tell my family that I believed I was dying, but also that I was dying from AIDS. I requested help to do this and AIDS Ministry became an important link to my family.

Although I didn't die, stabilizing my condition—physical and mental—was a slow process.

Recently I was asked what I thought pastors needed to hear, so I prepared this list of thoughts.

Through a friend, I know of the last days of a man who died this past week. Although I didn't know him, I have thought about him since his death. On his deathbed some of his final words were, "God is going to be angry—I'm gay and I am a murderer." This man was married and had not only denied who he was and the seriousness of his condition to himself, but had also denied these to his wife. These denials allowed him to continue his relationships— and his wife, angry and betrayed, has health concerns of her own now. I tell you this because for many people the issues and concerns are complex.

Know that the ones who get sicker and die faster might be those who continue to abuse their bodies and remain isolated in their anger, shame and denial. And the ones who give unconditional love and gain more acceptance of their condition and themselves from people also gain more peace and knowledge of how to care for themselves. This man had no power left to think healing thoughts because he had filled his mind with shame and anger.

Living with AIDS is a roller-coaster of health and emotions. It's living with a time bomb inside you—and no way of knowing when it will go off—so any little thing can become major in your mind. And it's about losing control over everything: money, health, actions and home.

AIDS also gives you perspective and changes your perceptions of all your relationships, whether physical, social or spiritual. We can measure our intimacy with God by our closeness to death. I will live until I die. We weren't meant to last forever. We are here for a very short time, whatever the amount, and death is the natural process.

People with AIDS need a focused, positive attitude. They need to be touched, they need to be accepted, they need anti-shame therapy.

When you realize you are sick, you are startlingly confronted with your mortality. To know you may soon feel the hand of God is a powerful thought, and causes you to take account of your life.

Dying people want to know that they are all right—not physically, but as a piece of the cosmic puzzle. They want to know that it's all right to journey on. And they want to know that they, how ever twisted their lives may appear, are forgiven.

STEVE KEN
ROLAND BI
LL DAVID·
LAWRENCE
JEFFREY·D
AVID MARK
CEASAR MICHAEL DAVID ROBERT DANIEL BILL
SCOTT EDUARDO ROBERTO ANGELO RONALD+
SUARVITO DONALD RICHARD LOYD BILL JULIE
SUSAN JEFF CARL KATHERINE CHRISTOPHE
R JAMES TERRY GRAHAM JOHN LANCE DONALD+
GLENN GERARD JEROME JOSEPH ALAN PETER+
JUAN KEIT
H GEORGE+
+GREGORY
LON PAULINE
JONATHAN+
LON LAURA
ALBERT JIM
BRIAN LARRY
MELVIN SAM
ANTHONY+
ARTHUR KEN
JACK MARY
CARMEN RO
BERT DONNI
WILLIAM J
OSEPH MARC
ALAN CARL
PATRICK G
LENN ELDRE
D THOMAS+
NEIL MICKEY
DOMINIC JOE
FREDERICK
JOHN STEPHEN

## A Parish Transformed

### He tells his terrible secret,
### and it loses some of its terror

*(Reprinted with permission from the Minneapolis* Star Tribune*)*

H E TRIED TO BECOME A PRIEST, a young man from Paynesville, Minnesota, with an exuberance to preach. But on the verge of ordination he found himself rejected. The grounds: homosexuality.

He then planned a long life of music and service to his church. And once more he experienced a form of rejection, not by the church but in a diagnosis from a doctor three years ago, the result of a test. It was stunning and it was irreversible.

But four days ago the choirmaster stood before a congregation of nearly 2,000 at St. Edward's Catholic Church in Bloomington and declared the truth of his life: He is gay, he has AIDS and he is dying. There was no trace of morbidity in his voice. He spoke buoyantly of his union with the people of the church and of the privilege of being their music man, and finally he asked:

"And you love me, too, don't you?"

It was an appeal. It asked for an affirmation. He had protected his secret life because he was afraid of more rejection. This one would have been the most devastating, from the congregation to which he had given his music for nine years.

The applause was instantaneous and electric.

It rolled through the church and swept over the altar, where Larry Gully stood in his navy blue suit and red silk tie and his mortality and—now in a waning hour of his life—the liberating light of his acceptance.

With the help of a nun he lit a large violet candle and asked the congregation to pray for him. From the rear of the hall the choir that was the culmination of his nine years of work with the church sang a mantra-like repetitive melody from the Taize religious community in France, music that Gully had introduced to the church.

A woman who attended the service as a visitor, unprepared for the scene, said it was one of the most astonishing moments of her life.

"There was such a tremendous power in the unity of the people and their desire to embrace this man," she said. It seemed like something coming out of the deepest and most timeless instincts of humanity.

For the 44-year-old choirmaster, it exorcised the pain and isolation and the weight of evasions reaching back nearly 20 years.

For the congregation witnesses, it revealed in the starkest and most intimate way the cleansing power of honesty. It was more. Here was a face-to-face meeting with their own mortality in the presence of a friend, so close to death yet full of spiritual vitality.

He wasn't totally solemn about it. He had a few light one-liners. But his message was that he'd had to lie to save his reputation and his work. He concealed his homosexuality and later, after he acquired AIDS, he explained the weight loss by telling friends that he had cancer.

In the 1970s, a month before he was to be ordained a priest at the seminary in St. John's University in Collegeville, Minnesota, he had told the bishop that he was gay.

"I told him I may as well be honest with him because it was too much a burden to carry that lie into the priesthood. I thought he responded beautifully. He was kind and he was a friend. He thanked me for my honesty but he said he had to serve the church and he couldn't approve my ordination."

Gully decided that he would serve his church with music. He obtained advanced degrees from St. John's and Catholic University and a doctorate in Munich, West Germany. He served as liturgist at St. Mary's in Little Falls and at St. Joseph's in New Hope in the mid- and late 1970s, and in 1980 joined St. Edward's, one of the largest Catholic churches in Minnesota, with a membership of some 6,000. He was innovative, effusive. Sometimes flamboyant, always motivated, sometimes bigger than life. Although some folks in the congregation were never going to write fan mail to Larry Gully, he acquired broad popularity for his energy and art, his willingness to please and his clear yearning to be liked. He assembled an exceptional choir and made St. Edward's a campus for diversified sacred music, from progressive, jazzy stuff to traditional and medieval.

Three years ago the doctor told him he tested positive for the AIDS virus. He told no one except his parents in Paynesville until a little more than a week ago, when his condition had declined to the point where the pastor and the church administrator met with him to talk about it. It was pointless by then, he decided, to extend the masquerade. He told them for the first time about being gay and having AIDS. "They couldn't have been better and more understanding about it," he said. "We thought it would be just as well if I told the congregation, because I was going to have to leave. The AIDS has reached that point where I needed more treatment. Last weekend was my last. I had begun to tell small groups within the church, and when the hour came to tell the congregation, I wasn't nervous at all. I was at peace."

Gully spoke four times to the membership, once Saturday night and three times Sunday morning. Each time the director of AIDS Ministry for the Archdiocese stood at his side and helped him to light the candle. In each case the pastor introduced him warmly by drawing from the morality play "Everyman," which makes the point that good works remain as a legacy in the lives of men and women after their wit, beauty and intelligence slip away. He thought that was a way to remember Larry Gully.

It was a tricky theological road for the church's hierarchy, which didn't want to be seen endorsing the gay lifestyle in giving Larry Gully a round-the-clock forum to make his farewells and to declare his truth. But the church and the church's music were inseparable conditions of his life. "He has meant much to our church," the chief pastor said Tuesday. "It is late in his life. It was right to embrace him with our love and our compassion."

So, with the nun at his side, Gully left his choral podium and walked to the altar to give the homily, fragile and balding but very much in the environment he wanted to say his farewell. He spoke of the pain of his earlier rejection. "It was so deep that I could not tell any congregation what I really was for fear you would reject me and no longer love me. I'm so sorry I didn't tell you sooner, but I was so afraid. For me, it's been a marriage. Like a marriage I have loved you through all the sacraments—baptism, confirmation and the others. We have done it all. We have built one of the largest choirs, and we have done it with class."

In one of the services a 15-year-old girl interrupted her reading to tell him how much he meant to the youngsters in church.

The applause rose from the tears and silence, and when Gully returned to his chorus the congregation sang its heart out.

It was a catharsis for thousands, among them Larry Gully, a recognition that the power that brings humanity together is so much stronger, if nourished, than the ignorance and fear that drives it apart.

It was back to another world yesterday for Larry Gully, seeing a doctor, taking medicines.

"Wasn't it beautiful?" he asked.

It still is.

*The following thoughts are from the pastor at St. Edward's Catholic Church where Larry Gully was the liturgist and music director.*

The parish administrator and I were the first to hear that Larry, our liturgist and music director at St. Edward's, wasn't dying of cancer. He was dying of AIDS.

Larry would no longer be leading us in music. We could face his homosexuality, his AIDS and his death. But we needed Larry's honesty to unite us so that we could face this loss together.

And so, with the encouragement from Sister Joanne Lucid, BVM, Director of AIDS Ministry of the Archdiocese of Saint Paul and Minneapolis, Larry decided to be honest with all the parishioners, to embrace his leaving and death with them. Larry shared his story with the parish staff, the pastoral council, the choir, and finally with the rest of the parish at the weekend Masses.

The guiding principle for that final sharing was helpful: keep it natural and simple. Larry did just that. He told the congregation he did not have cancer but was dying of AIDS and was gay. He asked for forgiveness for covering up the truth out of fear of rejection. He proclaimed his love for them and marveled over the music they made together. When he ended by lighting a candle, the congregation showed their compassion and affection for Larry with loving applause.

Larry's honesty challenged us. It demanded that our listening be free of judgment, and that we be compassionate while not condoning. It demanded that we face our own fears: of loss, homosexuality, AIDS and death. Professional counselors helped us sort through our thoughts and feelings.

Larry's honesty freed us to respond openly and genuinely. For forty-five days, volunteers cared for Larry around the clock, so that he could die in his own home. Others cleaned, cooked and supported his family, while still others wrote notes and made phone calls. And we all prayed. When Larry passed away in his condo, he was supported by the compassion and love of his family and the extended family he had created by his friendship.

God took our efforts and transformed us. Larry's Mass of Resurrection was joyful, natural and simple in a grand way because we had journeyed with Larry. We had faced the fears together and were victorious. We were a community of compassion and love through Larry's dying. Through Larry we could be as the Lord calls us: a people of the resurrection. Alleluia is the song we sing.

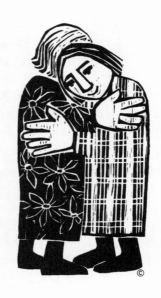

AIDS Ministry Program
The Archdiocese of Saint Paul and Minneapolis
Riverside Medical Center
Riverside at 25th Avenue, South
Minneapolis, Minnesota 55454
612/337-4345

# FOR THOSE WE LOVE

# Bibliography

The following bibliography, although extensive, is hardly all-inclusive. The medical literature alone is expanding exponentially. The books presented here are a taste of what is being written about AIDS from a variety of disciplines: medicine, psychology, sociology, journalism, law, pastoral care, and theology. The criteria for choosing these particular books were their usefulness for people with AIDS (PWA) and the impact that they made on the different disciplines mentioned above, as well as their availability to the general public. All of the books listed are readily available in local bookstores and libraries at the time of publication.

We have divided the bibliography into six categories:
- General Information About AIDS
- Psychosocial and Caregiving Issues in AIDS Work
- Gay People and Issues Related to AIDS
- Life's Spiritual Journey and AIDS
- Children, Youth, and AIDS
- Women and AIDS

Many of the books presented cross categories, but, it is to be hoped, you can see the rationale for categorizing them in this way. If there is a particular weakness in this bibliography, it is the paucity of sources on women and AIDS and on substance abuse in AIDS. It is only recently that substantial works in these areas have emerged.

Finally, it should be noted that many people will disagree with the choices we have made in this selection. Not everything will be equally appealing; the appropriateness of each work will depend on individual circumstances.

## I. General Information About AIDS

There are a variety of general information books on AIDS, everything from *Understanding and Preventing Aids* to the poignant stories found in Randy Shilt's journalistic account of the early days of AIDS, *And the Band Played On*. Some of the books, such as *The Truth About AIDS*, are dry reading, while others, such as Larry Kramer's *Reports from the Holocaust* and Paul Monette's *Borrowed Time: An AIDS Memoir*, are angry and impassioned. It is also important to check the date of publication when reading anything about AIDS, especially medical accounts, as new facts will often negate previous educated guesses. A lot of damage can be caused by incorrect or incomplete information.

Alyson, Sasha, ed. *You Can Do Something About AIDS.* The Stop AIDS Project. New York: Book of the Month Club, 1988. A public service project of the publishing industry.

Chirimuta, Richard, and Rosalind Chirimuta. *AIDS, Africa and Racism.* New York: Free Association Books, 1989.

de Saint Phalle, Niki. *AIDS: You Can't Catch It Holding Hands.* San Francisco: Lapis Press, 1987.

Fee, Elizabeth, and Daniel M. Fox, eds. *AIDS: The Burdens of History.* Berkeley: University of California Press, 1988.

Illingworth, Patricia. *AIDS and the Good Society: Points of Conflict.* New York: Routledge, Chapman, and Hall, 1990.

Jennings, Chris. *Understanding and Preventing AIDS.* Cambridge, Mass.: Health Alert Press, 1988.

Kramer, Larry. *Reports from the Holocaust.* New York: St. Martin's Press, 1989.

McCormack, Thomas P. *The AIDS Benefits Handbook.* New Haven, Conn.: Yale University Press, 1990.

McKusick, Leon. *What to Do About AIDS: Physicians and Mental Health Professionals Discuss the Issues.* Berkeley: University of California Press, 1986.

Monette, Paul. *Borrowed Time: An AIDS Memoir.* San Diego, Calif.: Harcourt Brace Jovanovich, 1988.

Nungesser, Lon G. *Epidemic of Courage: Facing AIDS in America.* New York: St. Martin's Press, 1988.

Price, Monroe E. *Shattered Mirrors: Our Search for Identity and Community in the AIDS Era.* Cambridge, Mass.: Harvard University Press, 1989.

Shilts, Randy. *And the Band Played On: Politics, People, and the AIDS Epidemic.* New York: St. Martin's Press, 1987.

Whitmore, George. *Someone Was Here: Profiles in the AIDS Epidemic.* New York: Grove Press, 1986.

———. *Someone Was Here: Problems in the AIDS Epidemic.* New York: NAL, 1988.

## II. Psychosocial and Caregiving Issues in AIDS Work

Of great importance to the caregiver is how AIDS affects the PWA's relationship with the rest of the community, family, friends, and coworkers. How does one cope with decreased ability to care for oneself, the loss of personal independence and power? How does the family cope with a disease that is physically devastating, emotionally taxing, and potentially shaming? How does one physically take care of someone with AIDS? How do you protect the person's rights?

The following books attempt to answer these questions. Some, such as *AIDS: A Health Care Management Response*, look at the whole health care system's response. Others, such as *An AIDS Caregiver's Handbook*, look at the primary caregiver's role in the psychosocial and physical care of the person with AIDS. Although the books suggested here deal specifically with AIDS, you should be aware that almost any book on chronic illness can be of help.

Altman, Dennis. *AIDS in the Mind of America: The Social, Political, and Psychological Input of a New Epidemic.* New York: Doubleday, 1987.

Blanchet, Kevin D. *AIDS: A Health Care Management Response.* Rockville, Md.: Aspen Publications, 1987.

Daley, Dennis. *Relapse Prevention: Treatment Alternatives and Counseling AIDS.* Human Services Institute. Blue Ridge Summit, Pa.: TAB Books, 1989.

Dietz, Steven, and M. Jane Parker Hicks. *Take These Broken Wings and Learn to Fly: The AIDS Support Book for Patients' Family and Friends.* Tucson, Ariz.: Harbinger House, 1989.

Dilley, James W., Cherry Pies, and Michael Helquist. *Face to Face: A Guide to AIDS Counseling.* AIDS Health Project of the University of California. Berkeley: Celestial Arts, 1989.

Dreurihle, Emmanuel. *Mortal Embrace: Living with AIDS.* Translated by Linda Coverdale. New York: Hill and Waring, 1988.

Eidson, Ted. *An AIDS Caregiver's Handbook.* New York: St. Martin's Press, 1989.

Greenly, Mike. *Chronicle: The Human Side of AIDS.* New York: Irvington, 1986.

Griggs, John, ed. *Simple Acts of Kindness: Volunteering in the Age of AIDS.* New York: United Hospital Fund of New York, 1989.

Hallman, David G. *AIDS Issues.* New York: Pilgrim Press, 1989.

Kirkpatrick, Bill. *AIDS: Sharing the Pain, A Guide for the Caregiver.* New York: Pilgrim Press, 1990.

Kubler-Ross, Elisabeth. *AIDS: The Ultimate Challenge.* New York: Macmillan, 1987.

McIlverna, Ted., ed. *Safe Sex in the Age of AIDS for Men and Women.* Secaucus, N.J.: Citadel Press, 1986.

Moffat, Betty Clare. *AIDS: A Self-Care Manual.* San Bernadino, Calif.: Borgo Press, 1987.

O'Malley, Padraic, ed. *The AIDS Epidemic: Private Rights and the Public Interest.* Boston: Beacon Press, 1989.

Perelli, Robert J. *Ministry to Persons with AIDS: A Family Systems Approach.* Minneapolis: Augsburg/Fortress, 1991.

Pohl, Mel, M.D., Deniston Kay, Ph.D., and Doug Toft. *The Caregivers' Journey.* Center City, Minn.: Hazelden, 1990.

Shelp, Earl E. *AIDS and the Church.* Philadelphia: Westminster, 1987.

____. *AIDS: Personal Stories in Pastoral Perspectives.* New York: Pilgrim Press, 1986.

Siegel, Larry. *AIDS and Substance Abuse.* New York: Harrington Park Press, 1987.

Sunderland, Ronald H., and Earl E. Shelp, *Handle with Care: A Handbook for Care Teams Serving People with AIDS.* Nashville: Abingdon Press, 1990.

Witt, Michael D., ed. *AIDS and Patient Management: Legal and Social Issues.* Owings Mills, Md.: National Health Publications, 1986.

## III. Gay People and Issues Related to AIDS

Much of the emotional pain surrounding AIDS stems from people's homophobia and from their misconceptions about gay and lesbian people that are translated into irrational hate and fear. Some of the following books, such as Mary Borhek's books on coming out and relating with a gay child, offer an insight into gay and lesbian issues in general, while Robert Nugent's *A Challenge to Love,* for instance, offers insights on maintaining self-worth in a hostile environment. All, however, challenge our general perceptions.

Borhek, Mary V. *My Son Erik*. New York: Pilgrim Press, 1984.

——. *Coming Out to Parents: A Two-Way Survival Guide for Lesbians and Gay Men and Their Parents*. New York: Pilgrim Press, 1985.

Delaney, Martin, and Peter Goldblum. *Strategies for Survival: A Gay Men's Health Manual for the Age of AIDS*. New York: St. Martin's Press, 1987.

Flood, Gregory. *I'm Looking for Mr. Right, But I Will Settle for Mr. Right-Away: AIDS, True Love, the Perils of Safe Sex, and Other Spiritual Concerns of the Gay Male*. Seattle, Wash.: Brob House Books, 1987.

Glaser, Chris. *Coming Out to God: Prayers for Lesbians and Gay Men, Our Families, Friends, and Advocates*. Louisville: Westminster/John Knox Press, 1991.

Grammick, Jeannine. *Homosexuality and the Catholic Church*. Mt. Rainier, Md.: New Ways Ministry, 1985.

Griffin, Carolyn, Marian Wirth, and Arthur Wirth. *Beyond Acceptance: Parents of Lesbians and Gays Talk About Their Experiences*. Englewood Cliffs, N.J.: Prentice Hall, 1986.

Nugent, Robert, ed. *A Challenge to Love: Gay and Lesbian Catholics in the Church*. New York: Crossroad, 1983.

Scanzoni, Letha, and Virginia Mollenkott. *Is the Homosexual My Neighbor? Another Christian View*. New York: Harper & Row, 1980.

# IV. Life's Spiritual Journey and AIDS

How does one maintain a sense of hope in the presence of chronic and terminal disease? How does one maintain self-esteem in the midst of shaming prejudice and fear? Where are our sources of strength in the midst of weakness? If one could say anything good has come of the AIDS epidemic, it would probably be in regard to the spiritual witness and growth that persons with AIDS and their families have shown—as well as in creative new uses for customary spiritual techniques. These range from the traditional (*AIDS: A Catholic Call for Compassion*) through meditations influenced by chemical dependency treatment programs (*The Color of Light: Daily Meditations for All of Us Living with AIDS*) and progressive spiritualities (*AIDS Book: A Positive Approach; Serenity*).

Badgley, Lawrence E. *Healing AIDS Naturally: Natural Therapies for the Immune System*. San Bruno, Calif.: Human Energy Press, 1987.

Bamforth, Nick. *AIDS and the Healer Within*. New York: Amethyst Press, 1987.

Bosnak, Robert. *Dreaming with an AIDS Patient*. Boston: Shambhala, 1989.

Bateson, Mary C., and Richard Goldsby. *Thinking AIDS*. Reading, Mass.: Addison-Wesley, 1988.

Boyd, Terry. *Living with AIDS: One Christian's Struggle*. Lima, Ohio: C.S.S. Publishing, 1990.

Callen, Michael. *Surviving AIDS*. New York: Harper & Row, 1990.

Flynn, Eileen P. *AIDS: A Catholic Call for Compassion.* Kansas City, Mo.: Sheed & Ward, 1985.

Fortunato, John E. *AIDS: The Spiritual Dilemma.* New York: Harper & Row, 1987.

Hay, Louise. *As Someone Dies.* Santa Monica, Calif.: Hay House, 1986.

_____. *AIDS Book: Creating a Positive Approach.* Santa Monica, Calif.: Hay House, 1988.

Iles, Robert H. *The Gospel Imperative in the Midst of AIDS.* Wilton, Conn.: Morehouse Publishing, 1989.

Kavar, Louis F. *Pastoral Ministry in the AIDS Era: Focus on Families and Friends of PWAs.* The Caregiver Series. Wayzata, Minn.: Woodland Publishing, 1988.

Keleman, Stanley. *Living Your Dying.* Berkeley, Calif.: Center Press, 1985.

Levine, Stephen. *Healing into Life and Death.* New York: Doubleday, Anchor Press, 1987.

Mueller, Howard E. *AIDS: A Christian Response (Study Guide for Adults).* St. Louis: Concordia Publishing House, 1988.

Oyler, Chris. *Go Toward the Light.* New York: Signet, 1988.

Reed, Paul. *Serenity.* Berkeley, Calif.: Celestial Arts, 1987.

Serinus, Jason, ed. *Psycho-Immunity and the Healing Process: A Holistic Approach to Immunity and AIDS.* Berkeley, Calif.: Celestial Arts, 1986.

Smith, Walter J. *Living and Dying with Hope: Issues in Pastoral Care.* Mahwah, N.J.: Paulist Press, 1988.

Snow, John. *Mortal Fears: Meditations on Death and AIDS.* Cambridge, Mass.: Cowley Publications, 1989.

Sunderland, Ronald H. *AIDS: A Manual for Pastoral Care*. Philadelphia: Westminster Press, 1987.

Tilleraas, Perry. *The Color of Light: Daily Meditations for All of Us Living with AIDS*. Center City, Minn.: Hazelden, 1988.

_____ . *The Circle of Hope: Our Stories of AIDS, Addiction, and Recovery*. San Francisco: Harper & Row, 1990.

## V. Children, Youth, and AIDS

As the AIDS crisis deepens we are becoming more aware of how it is affecting our children both as persons themselves with AIDS and their consciousness of the disease as it affects their lives. Slowly but surely an AIDS literature for children is appearing. What follows are a few books that address the subject of children with AIDS, tell us how to talk to children about AIDS, and are written for children to read about AIDS on their own.

Blake, Jeanne. *Risky Times: How to Be AIDS-Smart and Stay Healthy*. New York: Workman Publishing, 1990.

Cheik, William A. "AIDS." In *The Encyclopedia of Health: Medical Disorders and Their Treatment*, edited by Dale C. Garell, M.D. New York: Chelsea House, 1988. Primarily for mid to late adolescents.

Hausherr, Rosmarie. *Children and the AIDS Virus: A Book for Children, Parents, and Teachers*. New York: Clarion Books, 1989. To be read to grade-school children by adults.

Hein, Karen, M.D., and Teresa Foy DiGeronimo, eds.
*AIDS: Trading Fear for Facts: A Guide for Teens.*
Illustrated by Keith Haring. New York: Editors of
Consumer Reports, Consumers Union of the U.S.,
1989.

Kirp, David L. *Learning by Heart: AIDS and Schoolchildren in America's Communities.* New Brunswick, N.J.:
Rutgers University Press, 1989. For adults.

Madaras, Lynda. *Lynda Madaras Talks to Teens About
AIDS.* New York: Newmarket Press, 1988.

Marsh, Carole S. *Sex Stuff: A Book of Practical Information and Ideas for Kids 7–17, and Their Teachers
and Parents.* Bath, N.C.: Gallopade Publishing Group,
1987.

Merrifield, Margaret, M.D. *Come Sit by Me.* Illustrated by
Heather Collins. Toronto: Women's Press (517 College
Street, Suite 233, Toronto, Ontario M6G 4A2), 1990.
An education storybook on AIDS and HIV infection
for children 4-8 and their caregivers.

Quackenbush, Marcia, and Sylvia Villareal, M.D. *Does
AIDS Hurt? Educating Young Children About AIDS.*
Santa Cruz, Calif.: Network Publications, 1988.

Quackenbush, Marcia, and Mary Nelson, eds., with Kay
Clark. *The AIDS Challenge.* Santa Cruz, Calif.: Network Publications, 1988. Prevention education for
young people.

## VI. Women and AIDS

AIDS may have made its first appearances among the
male population, but it is a gender-blind disease. Less is

available about AIDS among women, as it has mostly struck the poor and disenfranchised, without voice—but the following resources will be helpful in speaking to the issues that uniquely address AIDS and women.

The ACT-UP/NY Women and AIDS Book Group. *Women, AIDS, and Activism.* Boston: South End Press, 1990.

Kaplan, Helen. *The Real Truth About Women and AIDS.* New York: Simon & Schuster, 1987.

Norwood, Chris. *Advice for Life: A Woman's Guide to AIDS Risks and Preventions.* New York: Pantheon Books, 1988.

Peavey, Fran. *Shallow Pool of Time.* Philadelphia: New Society Publishers, 1990.

Richardson, Diane. *Women and AIDS.* New York: Methuen. 1988.

Rieder, Innes, and Patricia Ruppelt, eds. *AIDS: The Women.* San Francisco: Cleis Press, 1988.

Watstein, Sarah Barbara, and Robert Anthony Laurich. *AIDS and Women: A Sourcebook.* Phoenix, Ariz.: Oryx Press, 1990.

# Directory of People, Places, and Other Resources

This is my experience as a person-living-with-AIDS. If someone wants to cook for me, clean for me, take me to dinner, bring me a present, I let them. Being diagnosed as having AIDS creates feelings of helplessness in people. It has become important to me to let other people into my life—including service agencies. I researched what services were out there, and I use the ones I need. I don't need all the services available that are offered, but I accept the ones I need right now. At first I rationalized that there are so many people who are worse off than I am and that I really didn't need any services. But I realized that accepting services from an agency whose purpose is to offer services to people with AIDS does not make me a victim or a "charity" case. I realized that it simply makes sense in all areas of life to take advantage of another person's expertise and experience. My outlook changed, and I found out that I, too, often had something to give to them. I felt better about myself as I helped myself. For me sometimes that means accepting help.

Where did I start? I checked out the resources listed in this small directory. I asked myself, "What are my needs? What do I want to know?" and made a list. I wrote down all my questions. "Is there a local organization of persons-living-with-AIDS/HIV in my area?" I asked my doctor. I used the national and state hotline entries. With other questions I called local pastors, regional church offices, AIDS Interfaith Network, state and county health departments, the United Way, the local Red Cross, the nearest university health care department, and city and state AIDS services. The groups are there to help me. When questions are complex, I ask to speak to the agency director or supervisor.

I do not have to go this hard road alone. I no longer isolate myself. I keep in touch and make contacts. There are times when this does not diminish the pain, but it helps me to know that others have felt confused, frightened, enraged, anxious, and in a panic. Now is the time for me to begin to build the future and to grow. I hope my suggestions will help you.

**Utilizing Support Resources**

People in your life are most effective when the support they provide fits their capabilities. Match your needs with the people who can best meet them. Avoid expecting people to give what they cannot. Remember that even the best support system will not be useful if you don't give it a chance to work. Let others know your needs and how they can help. Feel comfortable asking for support.

When should you ask for support? Anytime. Do not wait until after you've turned to food, alcohol, or drugs for support. Don't wait until your other relationships are suffering because of pressure. Especially don't wait until your own health suffers. Now is the time to seek support. It is there for you.

> Please Note: References were verified as of June 1991. In such a rapidly changing field, organizations and  hours of operation rapidly change. In the United States, use the National AIDS Hotline, your state hotline, or local resources for more assistance.

## UNITED STATES RESOURCES

### Hotlines

National AIDS Hotline
(800) 342–AIDS [2437]
Daily, 24 hours a day
> A free national hotline number for anyone with a question about AIDS. Also known as National HIV and AIDS Information Service. Respectful of privacy, with trained information specialists attuned to needs of callers. Directs callers to appropriate resources from more than 8,000 entries in its data base.

National Spanish AIDS Hotline
(800) 344–SIDA [7432]
Daily, 8:00 A.M. to 2:00 A.M. (EST)

National AIDS Hotline for Hearing Impaired
TTY/TDD (800) 243-7889
Monday-Friday, 10:00 A.M. to 10:00 P.M. (EST)

National Sexually Transmitted Disease Hotline
(800) 227-8922
Monday-Friday, 8:00 A.M. to 11:00 P.M. (EST)
    Referrals to public clinics, legal services, mental health
    resources, and others.

Project Inform
(800) 822-7422
Monday-Friday, 10:00 A.M. to 4:00 P.M. (PST);
Saturday, 10:00 A.M. to 1:00 P.M.
    Up-to-date information on treatment options.

## Resources

AIDS Ministry Program
The Roman Catholic Archdiocese of Saint Paul
    and Minneapolis
Riverside Medical Center
Riverside at 25th Avenue South
Minneapolis, MN 55454
(612) 337-4345
Daily, 24 hours a day
    Updated information on resources and referrals. Sup-
    port groups, volunteer training, retreats, and confer-
    ences.

AIDS Ministries and Programs
Division of American Missionary Association
United Church Board for Homeland Ministries
700 Prospect Avenue, East
Cleveland, OH 44115-1100
(216) 736-3270

AIDS National Interfaith Network (ANIN)
300 I Street, N.E., Suite 400
Washington, DC 20002
(202) 546-0807
Monday-Friday, 9:00 A.M. to 5:00 P.M. (EST)
   National coalition of local, regional, and national HIV/
   AIDS ministries. Resources for caregiving, education,
   and state and federal public policy advocacy. Up-to-
   date information about HIV/AIDS ministry networks
   in denominational and other religious bodies.

American Red Cross
Office of HIV/AIDS Education
1709 New York Avenue, N.W., Suite 208
Washington, DC 20006
(202) 662-1577
Monday-Friday, 8:30 A.M. to 5:00 P.M. (EST)
   Referrals and brochures.

   Regional offices:
      Midwestern Operational Headquarters
      (314) 997-3130
      Monday-Friday, 8:15 A.M. to 4:15 P.M. (EST)

      Eastern Operational Headquarters
      (703) 838-7766
      Monday-Friday, 8:30 A.M. to 4:45 P.M. (EST)

      Western Operational Headquarters
      (415) 375-7280
      Monday-Friday, 8:30 A.M. to 4:30 P.M. (PST)

   Write or call your local Red Cross chapter first, then
   the national office, then regional headquarters.

Federation of Parents and Friends of Lesbians
  and Gays, Inc.
P.O. Box 27605
Washington, DC 20038
(202) 638-4200
Monday-Friday, 9:00 A.M. to 5:00 P.M. (EST)
  Resources from AIDS Task Force for parents of HIV-
  positive gay men and lesbians.

HIV/AIDS Ministries Network
Health and Welfare Ministries Department
General Board of Global Ministries
United Methodist Church
475 Riverside Drive
New York, NY 10115
(212) 870-3871
Monday-Friday, 8:45 A.M. to 4:30 P.M. (EST)
  Focus papers, data bases, and information for churches
  and religious groups.

National AIDS Clearinghouse
PO Box 6003
Rockville, MD 20849-6003
(800) 458-5231
Monday-Friday, 8:30 A.M. to 7:00 P.M. (EST)
  Offers a wide variety of HIV/AIDS resources and
  referrals free of charge.

National Association of People with AIDS (NAPWA)
1413 K Street, N.W.
Washington, DC 20005

NAPWA *(continued)*
(202) 898-0414
Monday-Friday, 9:00 A.M. to 6:00 P.M. (EST)
    National 800 number given on request. Good monthly
    newsletter, *NAPWA News,* with features, regional
    updates, current drug protocol. NAPWA Link—a
    computer bulletin board and national speakers bureau.

National Coalition of Hispanic and Human Services
    Organizations (COSSMHO)
1030 15th Street, N.W., Room 1053
Washington, DC 20005
(202) 371-2100
Monday-Friday, 9:00 A.M. to 5:00 P.M. (EST)
    HIV/AIDS resources for the Hispanic community.

National Council of LaRaza
Union Center Plaza
810 First Street, N.E., Suite 300
Washington, DC 20002
(202) 289-1380
Monday–Friday, 8:30 A.M. to 5:30 P.M. (EST)
    HIV/AIDS resources for the Hispanic community.

National Minority AIDS Council
300 I Street, N.E., Suite 400
Washington, DC 20002
(202) 544-1076
Monday–Friday, 9:00 A.M. to 6:00 P.M. (EST)
    For referrals to organizations representing minority
    populations.

National Network of Runaway Youth
1400 I Street, N.W., Suite 330
Washington, DC 20005
(202) 682-4114
Monday-Friday, 8:30 A.M. to 5:30 P.M. (EST)
Resources for street youths, including those who are HIV-positive.

Shanti Project
525 Howard Street
San Francisco, CA 94105
(415) 777-CARE [2273]
Monday-Friday, 9:00 A.M. to 5:00 P.M. (PST)
Referrals to twelve other Shanti Projects spread out nationally and support groups and resources. Excellent volunteer training classes. Resource materials, movies, and pamphlets available.

## CANADIAN RESOURCES

AIDS Secretariat
Health and Welfare, Canada
Room 1750, Jeanne Mance Building
Tunney's Pasture
Ottawa, Ontario K1A 0L2
(613) 957-3069
Monday-Friday, 8:30 A.M. to 5:00 P.M. (EST)
Coordinates the National AIDS Strategy in collaboration with the department, other government offices, and key stakeholders. Organization is for groups, organizations, and institutions looking for information on programs, policies, and strategic directions.

Canadian AIDS Society
170 Laurier Avenue, West, Suite 1101
Ottawa, Ontario K1P 5V5
(613) 230-3530
Monday-Friday, 8:30 A.M. to 5:30 P.M. (EST)
  Organization composed of sixty community-based
  AIDS groups. Gives information on local and regional
  AIDS organizations that provide education, counsel-
  ing, information, advocacy.

Canadian Hemophilia Association
1450 Rue City Councilors, Suite 840
Montreal, Quebec H3A 2E6
(514) 848-0503
Monday-Friday, 8:30 A.M. to 4:30 P.M. (EST)
  Nonprofit health organization dedicated to improving
  the quality of life of persons with hemophilia and
  their families. Provides educational materials, peer
  support, research, and advocacy.

Canadian Public Health Association
National AIDS Clearinghouse
1565 Carling Avenue, Suite 400
Ottawa, Ontario K1Z 8R1
(613) 725-3769
Monday-Friday, 8:15 A.M. to 5:00 P.M. (EST)
  Central documentation center of AIDS education,
  prevention, and information materials. Distributes
  pamphlets; maintains lending library; compiles bibliog-
  raphies and reading lists.